PRAISE FOR *ZEN BENDER*

"I laughed and related to every page of this crazy mission to fix everything...that didn't need fixing. A wise, witty, and thought-provoking book that ends in just the place you'd hope it would. A great read whether you have a Reiki healer on speed dial, or, well, not."

—Marianne Power, author of *Help Me! One Woman's Quest to Find Out if Self-Help Really Can Change Your Life*

"Inspiring and hilarious, Zen Bender perfectly captures our misguided quest for perfection, as well as Stephanie's amazing spirit. I face the same daily struggles, so her writing really hit home with me, as I'm sure it will with everyone who has tried (and laughed about) all the fixes out there."

—Patricia Velasquez, actress on *Arrested Development* and *The Mummy*, author of *Straight Walk*, supermodel, and UNESCO Artist for Peace

ZEN BENDER

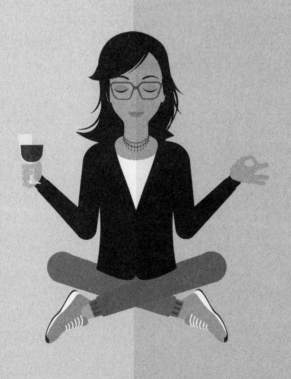

ZEN BENDER

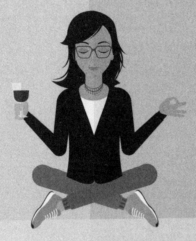

A Decade-Long Enthusiastic Quest to Fix Everything
(That Was Never Broken)

STEPHANIE KRIKORIAN

Mango Publishing
Coral Gables

Published by Mango Publishing Group, a division of Mango Media Inc.

Cover, Layout & Design: Morgane Leoni

Author Photo Credit: Erin Turner Photography

For permission requests, please contact the publisher at:
Mango Publishing Group
2850 S Douglas Road, 2nd Floor
Coral Gables, FL 33134 USA
info@mango.bz

For special orders, quantity sales, course adoptions and corporate sales, please email the publisher at sales@mango.bz. For trade and wholesale sales, please contact Ingram Publisher Services at customer.service@ingramcontent.com or +1.800.509.4887.

Zen Bender: A Decade-Long Enthusiastic Quest to Fix Everything (That Was Never Broken)

Library of Congress Cataloging-in-Publication number: 2019941762
ISBN: (print) 978-1-64250-029-5, (ebook) 978-1-64250-030-1
BISAC OCC010000, BODY, MIND & SPIRIT / Mindfulness & Meditation

Printed in the United States of America

This story is factually accurate to the best of my recollection. Still, at times, I've changed a name, or a situation, or been intentionally vague, so no story or conversation should be taken as exactly correct or that there is an exact person with the name given.

I'm also a truth seeker who goes out of my way to give credit where credit is due. My biggest panic when writing this book was that I inadvertently repeated an idea that I read somewhere else. Most of this book is what I have gleaned from my own experience. As you'll see from the pages you're about to dive into, I read and read and read and read a lot of articles on self-help and books on self-help. I've tried to give credit where due for thoughts that inspired me, but no one but me is responsible for the content of this book.

Stephanie Krikorian

TO JULIA AND DONALD KRIKORIAN FOR: EVERY. SINGLE.
THING. THIS GREAT LIFE OF MINE AND ALL OF ITS JOY IS
100 PERCENT THANKS TO YOU BOTH.

TO MY MOM'S LATE BROTHER, BILLY HARVEY, FOR THE
MOST IMPORTANT INTRODUCTION OF MY LIFE. WITHOUT
YOU, I MIGHT NEVER HAVE MET AND FALLEN FOR THE
BRIGHT LIGHTS OF THE BIG APPLE.

TABLE OF CONTENTS

NOTE TO READER

A *New York* magazine cover story in the summer of 2018, simply entitled *2008*, examined what's happened in the United States since the financial crisis, including a glossary of terms that have emerged as a result of the Great Recession. Along with *One Percent*, the *Sharing* and *Gig Economies*, *Millennials*, *Occupy*, and *Survivalism*, the term *Wellness* went mainstream.

The World Health Organization defines wellness as "a state of complete physical, mental, and social well-being." According to the Global Wellness Institute's website and various studies they have conducted, the global wellness industry was a $4.2 trillion market in 2018, up from $1.9 trillion in 2010.

While I was on my decade-long Zen Bender, I made a generous contribution to this sector.

PROLOGUE

When I look back at my childhood, I feel nothing but profound happiness and gratitude. My upbringing was simple and uncomplicated, but pleasant and warm, thanks to my parents.

My mom, Julia, was born to be a mom. My dad, Don, is a man of few words, but they are usually potent ones, with lessons buried within. Both have always been incredibly supportive.

When I told my dad at a young age that I was going to be an actress, something that many parents might find objectionable, he simply said, "First learn to waitress."

My dad was outnumbered. He (mostly) patiently put up with three yappy, opinionated, and strong-headed girls—Jackie (older), Jennifer (younger), and me in the middle. He carefully navigated our all-female household. Briefly, my dad had another guy in the house, my male tiger fish, Otto (I assumed he was male, not sure why). Otto was the only pet I ever had.

Rarely did my mom or dad interject in the bickering of the three of us. We were left alone to settle disputes on our own, probably in an effort to teach us to get along with other people later in life. While we didn't fight a lot, there were all-out wars over what we were watching on the television in our brown-wood-paneled rec room with wall-to-wall teal rug and textured plaster ceiling. Skilled at TV warfare, we would pull the knob off the wood-encased television set to prevent anyone else from changing the channel (long before TV's had remote control), thus preserving our viewing choice for as long as we wanted.

Jackie loved *Little House on the Prairie* reruns. I remember, vividly, walking in as she sat two feet away from the TV set, sobbing over

Laura Ingalls Wilder and family. Jennifer loved *The Love Boat*, and the soap opera *Santa Barbara*—the latter so much that she viewed the Capwells, the Lockridges, and the Castillos basically as family. I couldn't get enough of *Wonder Woman* and *The Bionic Woman*.

Eventually, of course, that knob used for changing the channel got lost, probably slipped down the side of the textured green-and-blue-striped couch. My father replaced it with a set of pliers that he set on top of the TV, but that required some seriously fine motor skills to hook onto the internal prong inside the broken channel-changing mechanism. He urged us not to lose them. We did not—they were too critical to our lives—but those pliers, in a pinch, doubled as a weapon when hurled across the room. Nobody lost an eye.

In the summers, we went on big camping vacations. To me, it always felt high-end, even though it was not. Even when camping, the lessons and skill-building continued. One in particular was in confidence, and lumberjacking, I suppose. My dad, much to my mother's horror, during a summer trip to Western Canada, handed me an axe at age eight, and offered me a few bucks to chop a big log in half. I did.

Later, with the cash stuffed into my blue and red patent-leather snap wallet, I stopped to fold T-shirts at the local tourist shop in Banff. Don't ask me why—I just did. Satisfied with my impromptu clean-up, I left the store, and my wallet and my cash behind. We all quickly ran back in; the wallet was there, but the money was gone. I was never big on folding laundry after that.

Every family has its own brand of humor, which might at times seem totally off the mark to other people. Ours was no different. When my sisters and I reminisce about the crazy things my dad used to say to us growing up, we always have a good laugh. We used to laugh when he said them back then, too.

When we were kids and we finished eating dinner, if we asked, "What's for dessert?" my dad would say, "Close your eyes."

We would.

"What do you see?" he would ask.

"Nothing," we would say, eyes closed.

"That's what's for dessert."

We eventually got savvy.

He taught me, in his own ultra-direct way, to "use my head" and think through a problem or a task. If I did something ultra-stupid, which I did from time to time, he would tell me with a chuckle, "For a smart girl, you're pretty dumb." (Prime example of us thinking something was funny while other people might think "Uh, child abuse.")

And there was his very unique way of teaching me the value of a dollar. Once, when I spent fifty dollars on a Ralph Lauren button-down denim shirt (which was on sale, half price, okay?), he told me I had "more money than brains." That sentiment has proven correct many times over.

Despite ours being an ordinary middle-class upbringing (my dad was a high school teacher and my mom a secretary), I didn't feel like I missed out on anything, not a toy or an outfit or an experience. I begged them to name my younger sister Ronald McDonald; that appeal was foolishly denied. But there was a Lite-Brite under the tree the year that it was the hot Christmas item, and a Cabbage Patch Kids doll named Ivy Marlene for me when they were all the rage (and people were fighting over them in the toy store). Everything was wrapped by my mother, so meticulously and perfectly; I have to this day never seen such professional wrapping skills.

One of my most vivid memories of sheer joy was when I was four or five and my dad drove up, home from work, and pulled a red, used, rusty bike from the back of the cream-colored VW camper. I watched as he walked it to me. It was mine. He had brought it home for *me*. My heart swelled with pride because he had gotten me something all my own, not for my birthday or Christmas, and not something that had once belonged to my older sister.

Of all the things I learned growing up, the one that started to ring in my ears later in life, was, perhaps, an early lesson in gratitude, not that I saw it as such then. Once, I desperately wanted a toy called a Lemon Twist. It was a black plastic cord that you attached to one leg, then whipped it around in a circle, repeatedly jumping over it with the other leg, while the lemon on the end swirled. I begged for it and eventually got it, but I remember my dad's initial response to my request.

"Why can't you just be happy you have two arms and two legs?"

Good question.

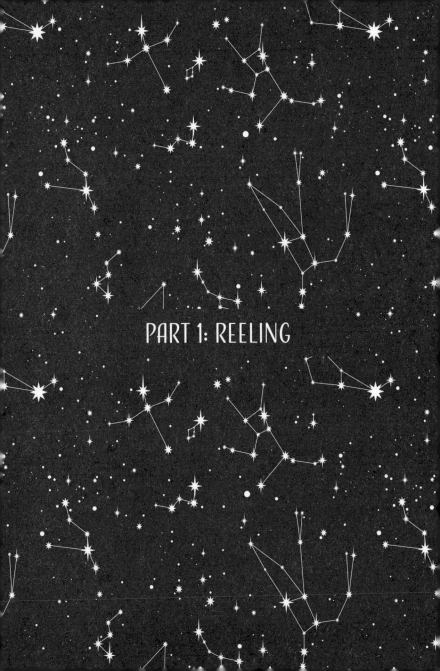

PART 1: REELING

MY GATEWAY DRUG: THE VISION BOARD

kaboom

I'm not going to say I quit a secure and well-paying job in news after working insanely hard to find it because of my vision board, but I'm not going to *not* say I did.

I'm kidding. I didn't.

Well, not really. But I did remain stalled at the intersection of Common Sense and the Universe (and all of its magic) for a long time while I debated my move. My career had ended, then it was briefly resuscitated. But it was hanging on by a thread, I knew that, so I needed to figure out what to do.

The Universe seduced me; the vision board was its Cyrano.

The vision board came into my purview around the time the book *The Secret* was picking up steam. Before I read it, I watched a discussion about it on *The Oprah Winfrey Show*, which was my church back then. When I watched Oprah and her guests talk about this book, I was transfixed. I had dabbled in yoga up until that point, but that was as New-Agey as I'd ever been.

The Secret was something different. It was out there, but not too out there. Out there in a way that made it make sense to at least consider its possibilities.

One practice *The Secret* made popular was the visualization notion upon which a vision board was based. Stare at a picture of a Ferrari, and soon enough, it will materialize. Its concept—that I could *will* something to happen with positive thinking—seemed interesting. Initially, I was mostly fascinated by the book's principle that, if you don't worry that a burger and fries will make you fat, *then it won't*, but scientific and exhaustive personal study had proven otherwise.

But this big idea: Letting go and allowing myself to be swept away by the power of an unseen force—that felt like something I could actually get behind. Jump, and the net will form.

People were anxious to cede control in order to get control of whatever was spiraling in their own lives. It was an interesting contradiction, but *The Secret* was, in a way, an adult magic wand.

And it, and all the self-help and spiritual books that followed, gave us all something to do.

I wasn't alone in pondering all that *The Secret* was offering up. The book became a pop culture phenomenon. It brought self-help and spirituality to the masses, perhaps thanks to Oprah, perhaps based on our need to believe. Years later, *Goop* picked up where Oprah and early adopters of the Universe and alternative fixes left off, blowing the lid right off the wellness market, making putting jade eggs in one's vagina basically conventional practice.

The Secret was a moment in time, a defining one indeed, that put what I called hocus-pocus into the mainstream.

All that I learned from that book initially got tucked away in that part of the brain that is filled with seemingly useless information that occasionally comes in handy at random times. I went on my merry, non-spiritual way and on to absorbing whatever else Oprah was talking about.

Any Self-Help Port in a Storm

It started out innocently enough. Right around the time things sort of got tough. That's often when and why we seek out self-help, because in a way, it's comfort food for our spirit. It's a life preserver when nothing else seems to help. Looking back, that's why I was drawn in.

At 10:30 a.m. on October 31, 2008, my career fell victim to the Great Recession. I was a news producer and journalist and had been working as such for almost eighteen years. After graduation from college, I wrote for a small newspaper, and then, after a year off for graduate school, dove straight into TV news. Until that fateful day when the show I worked on was abruptly canceled.

A year after I lost my job, I found another—albeit less exciting—one, but the damage had been done. "Frayed" would probably best describe my state of existence then. Initially, solace came in an interesting form: that vision board made popular by *The Secret* a couple of years earlier.

Desperate to find my way back to wherever it was that I was supposed to be, on the back of the steel door in my Harlem apartment, I made a very ad hoc, not-exactly-perfect-in-execution, first-timer's vision board. I didn't put a lot of back into it, to be honest—just slapped a few pictures up there, hoping for the best.

On that board, in full view, I used magnets to hang a cutout magazine picture of two Adirondack chairs with pretty pink pillows on them, facing out at a body of water (a.k.a. my future beach house that I would own because *renting* one wasn't enough), and a sleek city co-op that was, in my head and on my board, one hundred blocks downtown from the marble-countered, Kohler-fauceted two-bedroom I had just bought uptown. A tear sheet of a handsome male eyeballed me from the back of that door. He was my future husband. And a fit and thin woman working out was never going to be me, but a girl can be delusional, and staring at a skinny person would most definitely make me one, too. Right? Obviously, there was picture of a stack of cash, which I figured I needed to make all of the above materialize.

My vision. My perfect life, as told through magazine cutouts.

It was my starter vision board, the first time I had made one. (I'd later go on to make more.) At the time, I didn't know it, but I had a stronger vision-board game in me; this vision board was just a surface-scratcher.

Still, I believed that staring at those pictures every day as I left the apartment would surely make them a reality and therefore improve my life dramatically. It was easy to believe.

Believing in unseen forces, of course, meant ignoring that nagging and logical voice in my head that had always served me well. But then, if I could suddenly blame the Universe for a poor life decision when things got tough, I most certainly didn't have to blame myself.

AFOG (ANOTHER FUCKING OPPORTUNITY FOR GROWTH)

There was, of course, more to my frayed self than just the end of my career. That same year, I was also about to turn forty. Plus, I was *still* single. My middle section had gotten a little thicker than it had been in the past. Like rosé in the Hamptons in August, self-doubt was pouring non-stop into my head.

As my career came to a screeching halt and forty was looming, it increasingly felt like I was walking through waist-deep mud, slowly, unable to get anywhere. Stuck. As I struggled to gain my footing on all fronts, I wondered why everything *almost* but never quite seemed to happen for me. I worked hard not to compare my life to others', but I started to feel like I was on the local train and everybody else was on the express.

The problem was that, while I desperately craved a map to somewhere, I didn't know where exactly that was.

Eventually, my New Age and self-help efforts went next-level. It wasn't difficult. All I had to do was open my eyes, read a magazine, or listen to a talk show. Suddenly, everywhere I looked there was another fucking opportunity for growth. AFOG.

The Secret had ratcheted things up a few notches. This stuff was fully and readily available. Plus, we were in an economic downturn, and people were feeling desperate. Where does one turn when feeling desperate? Self-help. If you couldn't find a job, you could always self-improve. That was, after all, my first instinct.

It was not the job market, or the dating pool, or my weight—it was me. There was something wrong with me. There had to be. Which meant self-help books were suddenly the macaroni and cheese of comfort. The world had made a few things in my life feel out of control, so rather than sitting still, I chased a fix.

Like flashing neon signs on the Vegas Strip, the vision board had actually highlighted my shortcomings until, eventually, all I could see were the holes. Apparently, the Universe wasn't just offering up beach houses. It was offering up a full roster of experts, happy to sell you the way to a better life. Suddenly, self-help began screaming my name, which meant that, despite already having a great life by most measures, I wasn't maxing out my greatness.

Oprah created a mantra: "Live your best life." Which surely meant I wasn't living mine. None of us were, presumably. Just a big world full of humans not living up to our potential. All I saw was everything about myself that couldn't possibly have been as good as it needed to be. And so—just like a bag of chips—I assumed that, if all those fixes were sitting right there in front of me, then I should most definitely be consuming them. Not doing so seemed downright irresponsible. Or, at least, insulting to Oprah.

Eventually, I decided that if I kept reading more and hiring more coaches and trying new diets I'd 100 percent find not only the map, but also the destination.

And so, for nearly a decade, I went on a high-speed chase with balance, enlightenment, growth, and betterment—over-guruing myself with near desperation in an effort to be the absolute best I could be. I hit the healer circuit hard, like it was my job. It was a noisy ten years that resulted in a couple of major, off-the-rails Zen Benders, but not for one second did I declare a cease-fire between me and the urge to fix me.

Until I finally did. And certainly not in the way, or for the reason, that I would have expected.

A Far-from-Exhaustive List of What I Was Told and Sold on the New Age and Self-Help Circuit

From the Dating Coach: Always wear high heels on a date, and keep the first date to one hour.

From the seminar on *Why I'm Single*: Keep hair long and shiny to show you're fertile. Then someone will want to marry you.

From the Life Coach: Make a vision board, but don't overload it with too many hopes and dreams (like I did on my second and third vision boards). Wish a little smaller and tighter, or the big-ticket items will not happen.

From the *other* Life Coach: Write yourself a check for a million dollars and look at it every day. Eventually, you'll be successful and rich, and able to cash that check. (Still waiting.)

From the Rainbow Healer: You work too hard and nothing is ever good enough because you want to be liked because you must have been traumatized as a child. (I was not.)

From the Acupuncturist: You keep weight on to make yourself larger to keep people away—to literally create more space between them and you. (I'm a New Yorker. I like my space.)

From the Alternative Medicine Practitioner: If you sleep with a $150 magnet on your foot (magnetic therapy) when you have an injury, it will heal you. Unless, well, it won't. Especially if what you really need is foot surgery to remove a three-inch piece of wood from your foot. Like I did. (True story.)

From the Spa: Squat bare-assed over burning incense at a high-end hotel. (I'm not sure what that was supposed to do, but it was expensive, so I assumed it couldn't be bad.)

From Everybody Every Day: Beware of Mercury in retrograde. Don't sign contracts during this time. (And, uh, trust me, your lawyer and your clients won't think you're nuts when you delay executing a deal for a week. Or at least they won't tell you.)

From a Clairvoyant: Smudge your house with smoldering dry sage to get the bad juju out. (Feels like you're doing something even if you're not.)

From a Supermodel: Be sure to keep a cactus, and if it dies figure out who was at your house, because someone bad killed it by being there. (I did that. And a cactus died once. So, I moved. Not 100 percent because of the dead cactus, but I couldn't remember who had killed it and I hadn't yet learned how to smudge the place.)

From a Book: Dyeing a red streak in your hair will lead to personal and creative achievement, like *The Artist's Way* said it would. (It said to do something wild that you wouldn't normally do, and for me, wild meant a red streak.)

From Marie Kondo: Throw out all clothing that doesn't spark joy. (This will mostly leave you with nothing to wear.)

From the Feng Shui Police: Put flowers to the right side of your desk if you want to find love. Put something green to the left so that you'll get rich. Put reminders of your accomplishments in the center to ensure that you accomplish more. (Still waiting on said promised results.)

From a Random Magazine: Write negative things down on slips of paper and put them in the freezer every year to clear them away. (Or end up with a freezer full of stickies.)

On the other side of the Great Recession of 2008, there were those stories of the people who prevailed and happily came up with a second act, built million-dollar businesses, and overcame the big layoff during what felt like the end of days. There was also the flip side of that coin: the heartbreakers about the people who never recovered, who lost their homes and livelihoods, and experienced insurmountable declines in health.

My layoff wasn't like any of these. It wasn't as dramatic, or nearly as dire. I had enough friends and family in my life to know I'd never be homeless or hungry. They were all incredibly generous, keeping the wine flowing and, in my mom's case, the health-care premium paid for. But it still stung.

And, unlike the fog Valium gives you the day after you take it, the burden and anxiety of my layoff never, ever left me. I don't wish job loss on anybody. Even as a layoff based on the economy and not my performance, it felt deeply upsetting and utterly personal. Not to mention painfully embarrassing.

This book certainly isn't another the-recession-hit-then-I-found-a-job story. I don't want to dwell on the job loss here, but it was, as they say in the movies, the inciting incident. And while it consumed me for a long time, I finally realized, it's not *the* story, just a tiny part of this one.

Still, here's the way it played out...

THE END OF EVERYTHING

survival

In mid-September 2008, Lehman Brothers collapsed, and things were looking bleak across the country. That was putting it mildly. We were staring into a global economic abyss. At the time, I was producing a television show for *BusinessWeek* magazine called *BusinessWeekTV*. It was a financial news show produced on the forty-ninth floor of the McGraw-Hill building, so we were keenly aware of what was happening, economically speaking.

Right around that time, my friend and colleague Wendy and I were running out to grab lunch. As we waited for the elevator, we ran into Jack, the guy who did the budgets. Jack being a usually chatty and friendly person, we asked how he was, and he explained that he was frazzled because it was budget time and he was working long days.

Friendly and amusing as always, Wendy said to him, "Make sure you leave enough for us in TV."

If there was an Academy Award for Best Worst Poker Face, Jack would have won it. He froze. His smile vanished and his face went white. Then he practically dove headfirst into the elevator without saying a word.

Wendy and I looked at each other after he left and noisily burst out laughing. "Well, that was awkward," she said. We thought perhaps there would be some belt-tightening—no more holiday dinners at Bobby Van's. Maybe due to lack of imagination, or over-confidence, or just plain naiveté, we had no idea what we were in for.

We should have known better.

Still, I didn't think too much of Jack in the elevator. Later, I was meeting some friends for dinner at Otto off Fifth Avenue, and I had some time to kill. As usual, I was ultra-early, so I sat on a bench and stared at the fountain in that little triangle park where Bleecker Street and Sixth Avenue intersect.

I had a bad feeling that I couldn't shake, so I called the anchor of our show as I sat there soaking in the last licks of September sunshine.

"Do you think we will lose our jobs?"

She insisted we had nothing to worry about because we were making money for the company. Still, deep in my gut, I felt a shift on the horizon.

And, of course, there was the Jack incident, this probably marked the last time for a long time that I would trust my gut.

When in Doubt, Buy a Bad-Ass Handbag

Anticipating that I might never again earn a proper living, I did what everyone should *never* do when facing unemployment and financial collapse. I got up from my seat in that park and walked, with urgency, to Marc by Marc Jacobs and bought a show-stopping five-hundred-dollar purple leather bag.

It was a floppy, large, chunky-hardware, hobo-type bag with lots of outside pockets (a subway rider's dream). For years, I'd been contemplating what life would be like if I owned that bag or one like it, but up until then I'd never spent five hundred dollars on any single clothing item or accessory. It was an insane purchase, but I felt strongly it was the last expensive purse I'd ever be able to afford. I joked later that night with my friends that if I did get laid off, I would live in the handbag.

I had been right to worry.

A week later, I was late to work. Very late, for some reason I can't remember. At ten fifteen, I got a call from my boss asking where I was. I said I was on my way in a cab. He'd never called before.

"Hurry up and get here," he said. "We're all assembled in the conference room."

"Are we being laid off?" I asked. Somehow I knew.

"I can't say," he said.

"So, yes," I said.

I was late for my layoff.

Everyone had been sitting in the conference room since nine, waiting to get axed, when I rolled in wearing ripped jeans and black suede boots suitable for farming. They had filed out eventually, and when I finally arrived everyone filed back in. And with a prepared statement and limited information from non-human human resources types, it was over.

The magazine would live. The TV show and my career would die.

I was gutted. In slow motion, everybody on the team walked to their desks and made a phone call. I didn't call anybody right away. I just sat there and stared off into space, feeling humiliated. I'd never experienced anything like this before, and I simply didn't know what to do.

Later that day, on the subway ride home, I looked at all the people on the B train heading uptown and wondered if they knew I was a loser, who, in three months' time, would be without a paycheck.

"This will be the best thing that ever happened to you." I heard that a lot from well-meaning friends when, shell-shocked, I told them what had happened with my job.

I'll say this as yogically and New-Age-ily as I can, but every single time someone said that to me after I was laid off, as a single-income homeowner facing a mortgage on a two-bedroom apartment in New York City, staring at the end of my thirties—and likely the end of my best days professionally, not to mention for my ovaries—I wanted to literally punch the living crap out of them.

And I've never hit anybody. Except my younger sister, Jennifer, but only once, and that was a long time ago.

Even now, after making it through the layoff, I don't view my experience as "great" or "the best" in any way. To be very clear: Getting laid off was not at the time, nor is it viewed by me today as, the best thing that ever happened to me. Not even close.

Getting a coupon for a free bagel and cream cheese in a gift bag at a charity event was a better, more enjoyable life event. Losing my American Express card somewhere on 72nd Street, then replacing it, only to have the new card fall out of my pocket again two weeks later—basically sprinkling Manhattan with my line of credit but *having nobody use either card*—was a more thrilling life event than getting laid off.

In fact, rage was all I felt when that sentiment was recklessly tossed my way by well-meaning friends. To this day, I don't view it as the best thing that ever happened to me, but the worst, maybe. And I concede that, if that's the worst thing that ever happened to me, I'm an incredibly fortunate person.

Did I get through it? Yes. Over it? No. Not even close.

Only looking back do I see where that sentiment may have come from. They'd all been watching Oprah, too.

The Secret had permeated the collective mindset by that point. Many people were suddenly and breathlessly explaining to me that I could finally "do what I loved!" with my life. (I, by the way, loved working in television news.)

There they were, the first squeaks of self-help-esque optimism. Most everybody seemed gung-ho and on board with the Best Thing attitude. Keep in mind, I was a product of the '90s workforce. Work-life balance? What the fuck was that? You worked. Period. I am the daughter of parents who worked every day to provide for their children and the granddaughter of an

Armenian immigrant named Mgerdich Krikorian, who walked to work to pour steel in the foundry for a dollar a day so he could send his four children to school. Doing what you loved? Liked, maybe.

Of course, this sentiment was coming from people with paychecks and spouses with paychecks and 401ks and health care—people who were all fine espousing the new-found New Age wisdom, but I don't recall too many of them leaving their six-figure jobs to practice what they were preaching. There's a chance that the concept of facing what I was facing seemed a dream to them. Perhaps they were seducing themselves to not have to decide to leave a job they didn't like and chase a dream? Maybe. Maybe they really did see me as the lucky one.

Still, what New Age way of thinking could possibly suggest that an end to a career that I loved was the best thing? Or was I being too pessimistic in my frustration? Would my mortgage company in fact take a check for "doing what I loved," or did that require actual money?

Something else that I found weird at that time that always stuck with me: Many people felt the need to point out that things could have been worse. We all knew that. Things can always be worse. It was true.

But it's not exactly the thing you need or want to hear as you face your own personal end of days.

"At least you don't have cancer."

I didn't. And for that I was grateful. But that didn't mean my crisis was any easier on me.

One person said it was hard to feel sorry for me because I had so much going for me. Again, the cable company wasn't taking checks for "stuff I have going for me."

Plus, there was almost a hierarchy of pity surrounding a city of laid-off people. Many people talked about how badly they felt for "breadwinners"—a.k.a. men with families who had to feed their children and put them through private school. As a single and childless woman with a mortgage, just FYI, I was, and continue to be, the breadwinner in my home, too.

It was like an onslaught of weird advice that Lucy from Peanuts gave to Charlie Brown from her psychiatric booth, and at the time, I simply wasn't in the mood for, or buying into, it.

Not quite yet anyway, though I was soon to be born again myself.

All the sentiment led to some layoff takeaway that probably goes against the grain of most self-help thinking: Nobody wants to hear the easy-to-offer hypothetical bright side when they are drenched in self-pity and drowning in uncertainty. I did not. I just wanted to soak in my own agony for a while, so I could feel it, and sort through my personal crisis, however great or small it was to someone else; I wanted to acknowledge the pain of it all before taking action to fix it.

Perhaps friends, or society, or whatever we are collectively, don't want to deal with the discomfort of such a situation. But, looking back, avoiding the struggle that I was feeling wasn't the answer. Not for me. And not now that I've gone through it.

My advice today? When a friend is having a hard time, let her cry it out. Acknowledge: *This sucks*. Feel it with her. Don't skimp on agreeing. Tell her, "You have every right to be upset. Take a few days, eat potato chips for breakfast. Stay in your pajamas and watch back-to-back *Law & Order* repeats. (I have heard that that is a thing...from, uh, a friend.) Feel the sting. Don't avoid it or look for the sunny side until you're ready."

Nobody in crisis needs to hear that it could be worse.

Nobody needs to hear that their anxiety isn't worthy of a sob fest.

IRRATIONAL PANIC

In the months that followed getting laid off, I went on thirty-one job interviews. It was a challenging time. It felt like musical chairs. There were jobs, then a chair was pulled away and there were fewer options out there.

People were rapidly getting laid off, dropping like flies. This led me to face the realization that returning to a position in television news, at a certain level on the ladder, was going to be even more of a challenge than I'd thought when the hammer first came down.

I remember a former colleague named Peggy called me the afternoon we'd all gotten the axe because she'd heard about the cutbacks. She connected me with people at her network, and within days, I went in for an interview. I was feeling optimistic. For like five minutes. After lots of initial enthusiasm, I didn't hear anything back. Why? They had all gotten laid off, too. That didn't happen just once. It was like dominos at that time, and I was struggling to get out in front of it.

I went for four interviews at a major cable network for a single job. It was a job that I had been qualified for a decade earlier, but still, it was a job and, as my mother might have said, beggars can't be choosers. It was a morning-show gig and I had done my homework. By the time the fourth and final job interview came around (which meant four different outfits, a stressor for me, by the way), I had spent the week watching the show and charting the segments they had aired. I recorded the competition each day and did the same there, then I compared everything and made notes on each network's choices and what I might have done differently had I been producing.

I felt ready to take on that final interview, prepared, fully versed on the news of the week, the anchors of the show, and more.

When, halfway through the interview, one of the anchors asked me if I had watched that day, and what I might have done differently had I been producing, I was immediately thrilled because I *had* watched and I had several suggestions. Then I panicked. I couldn't remember a single thing. It had not crossed my mind to bring my pages of notes into the meeting.

My mind was suddenly empty.

Nerves frayed from the trauma of studying, finding new things to wear, and making sure I sounded like I knew what I was talking about, I blanked.

Full. On. Blanked.

And suddenly so frantic was I that recovery was 100 percent impossible.

"I did watch," I said to the room full of people awkwardly waiting to hear, "but I can't remember anything right now."

It was all the more tragic because it sounded like every unemployed producer on the planet had applied for that job, and as I understood it, it was down to the final two, me being one. I stumbled through the rest of my interview, mortified and humiliated, and after I left, I didn't make it out the door of that building before bursting into tears.

I was buckling under the pressure of the search.

But the Universe must have had plans for me. What was it telling me? That was very unclear.

Once it became painfully obvious that a real job wasn't going to happen fast, and once I learned what severance-plus-unemployment-plus-subsidies-from-my-mom were going to look like and how grim the job market was, I made a budget and instituted my own austerity program.

Molton Brown soap was sadly the first indulgence to go. Ivory bar soap would do just fine. All subscriptions to magazines and newspapers went away too—canceled immediately. Instead, the nail salon downstairs in my building served as a de facto library, and I would go and sit there to find out which stars were, in fact, *just like us*. I snatched my neighbors' discarded newspapers, and I curated a list of user logins from friends for major newspapers online and premium TV channels. Pride went out the door.

I initiated a one-pump rule for all remaining soap-like products—shampoo, conditioner, face wash, and moisturizer. No more mindlessly pumping a handful of liquid; I was on a budget. Every once in a while, when I was feeling blue or neglected, I'd hesitantly treat myself to a second pump. I stopped taking cabs. I stopped taking classes.

I sold some stuff, including a pole-dancing pole I had installed in the second bedroom. I had jumped on the popular pole-dancing-class bandwagon (to feel empowered, I was told). Class was super fun and physically challenging, but while most people could climb to the top of the pole in class, I found I could not. I would slide down and not be able to do the flip at the top—or all the good moves that came with hoisting oneself to the ceiling.

I didn't feel empowered, I felt pissed-off. So, I bought a pole and had it installed in my apartment so I could practice climbing at home. Competitive much? (I never made it to the top. Not once.)

So, along with fancy soap, I said goodbye to the pole and the pricey classes that went with it.

Shopping was no longer an activity for me either, unless it was mission-critical. I canceled my gym membership and the trainer, too. For the first time in my life, I priced out items like toilet paper and paper towels, and almost daily did a cash tally, measuring out just how far I could stretch things if the worst happened and I found no work.

In hindsight, I perhaps unnecessarily catastrophized the situation. And to this day, I'm a catastrophizer, thanks to the worry of not having a regular paycheck.

I braced for the worst.

My severance ran out on March 27, 2009, and that was a more brutal day than the layoff itself. That's when hope died and panic set in.

When I went on unemployment, as per some official New York State policy, I had to go downtown to a state-run resume seminar. I won't lie: I was heading in there with serious attitude. I couldn't believe I had to endure the humiliation of learning to make a resume. Uh, I got this. I don't need a seminar. I wanted to spend the time looking for jobs. But, to my surprise, my irkedness paled in comparison to the rest of the crowd. My class was filled with Wall Street guys whose body language (arms crossed, no pen in hand, slouched down in their seat) made clear they were more pissed-off than I was to be there. They were wearing super fancy watches, beautifully tailored untucked striped shirts, and expensive sunglasses propped on top of their heads. And they weren't happy. I realized then that, while my job loss sucked bad, they had further to fall than I did, financially speaking. It's a long drop from a healthy seven figures to unemployment. I wondered what their austerity budgets looked like. I was giving up expensive hand soap. They were giving up second and third homes. Still, like the entire process, it was emotionally draining and completely demoralizing.

The professional trauma hit me hard. In fact, for many years, it was the driving force behind many of my life decisions. But, instead of assessing the circumstances around me that may have contributed, I looked inward: *Here's what's wrong with you, and that is why you are here*.

It took a decade to realize that landing thirty-one interviews in an employment crisis was an impressive feat. But, at the time, I didn't know that. It didn't feel impressive.

It felt desperate.

YOU CAN EAT YOUR DINNER OR DRINK YOUR DINNER, BUT YOU CAN'T DO BOTH

career

For one hot second, being a little chubby paid off. In fact, it was the impetus for career number two.

My battle with my weight started in my mid-twenties. Once I was introduced to the adult world of working all day, the culinary thrill that is New York City, and traveling and therefore eating out on a corporate card, a never-ending war with the scale began. I was a skinny enough kid, but as an adult, my weight could best be described as up and down like a toilet seat at a party. It probably always will be, try as I may to manage that struggle.

I had done some radical diets over the years, but pre-layoff, around 2006 or 2007, I decided to see a registered dietician on a weekly basis. As part of her process, I would write down my food in a journal each week and track my calories, a startling and painfully revealing exercise.

Did you know a Starbucks Vente skim latte has about 130 calories?

A quarter of an avocado has 100.

Each week, when I had my appointment, I had to show the nutritionist what I had been taking in. She had a lot of funny lines, including, after seeing my notes listing margaritas (plural) with a platter of Mexican food, "You can either eat your dinner or drink your dinner, but you can't do both."

Translation: If losing weight when you are on the south side of five foot two means consuming 1350 calories per day, not per meal, then using 500 or, okay, 750 of them on three drinks is problematic.

After hearing that particular line, I told her she should write a book. She told me she didn't know how to write a book, so I trotted down to Barnes & Noble and bought a book on how to write a non-fiction book proposal to see if I could drag a book out of her. We teamed up, found an agent (Maura, still my agent today), and actually sold the proposal for *Urban Skinny*!

I still had my job at *BusinessWeek* at the time, so collaborating on a book was just what kids today call a side hustle.

Though I wrote that book while I was still employed, it wouldn't hit the shelves for years, after I'd been laid off.

Broken and Breaking Free

After the thirty-one job interviews, seven months into my layoff, I did eventually get some challenging, albeit low-paying, full-time freelance work at the *Wall Street Journal,* developing and launching their live digital programming. It paid less than half of what I was making when I was laid off at *BusinessWeek,* but it truly was a blast. The people I worked with were clever, young, and entrepreneurial in a way I'd not experienced.

We were a good team, too—Lauren Goode and Kelly Evans and the crack-of-dawn shift that left us delirious. Despite the criminally early call time, we had some seriously good laughs, once with Kelly over my lack of even a basic understanding of how to make an Excel spreadsheet (I still have no clue), and frequently over an obsession Lauren and I had with some moisturizing hand lotion called Glysomed that you can only buy in Canada.

Five months later, a full year after getting laid off, I was finally offered two full-time, semi-interesting jobs, with benefits, in news. One was a continuation of my gig at the *Wall Street Journal,* and one involved doing something similar at Reuters.

Both were digital programming, not television per se. Of the two jobs, I had to take the Reuters one. It excited me the least but paid the most. It was a financial necessity, not a choice.

Anti-*The Secret*? Yes.

Pro-avoiding going broke? Also yes.

While I was grateful, and it was a tremendous relief to finally have the illusion of job stability, as I faced starting a new gig in my humbled and traumatized state, I knew it would be difficult. The simple reality was that I was gun-shy; my confidence had been broken. My half-assed vision board had done nothing to change that. I was visualizing the shit out of life, but mostly I was just worried that, no matter where I worked, I wouldn't succeed.

Starting a new job is hard under any circumstances. It takes months before you know where the photocopier is, who is nice and who is not, how to change the way you work to fit a different culture than you might have experienced at a previous job. It's hard to hit your stride at any job, let alone one you took out of desperation.

That job, that I had scrambled to land, that I went on thirty-one job interviews to find, was, at the very least, ill-fitting. Not only was it not what I would have chosen, but it didn't feel like a productive or positive environment for a million reasons. And that added to my overall anxiety.

I knew five days into it that it was a bad fit. It wasn't actually television. And, while the people I worked with were unquestionably the most dedicated and fun group of journalists I'd ever had the pleasure of working with, the job itself just was not for me.

Which brings me back to the vision board.

Just as I was deep in the throes of hating my new, not even one-year-into-it job, I joined up with a group of creative and like-minded women who had, by choice or by way of the recession, started working for themselves, all while trying to find their way in the murky waters of a new economy. Some had turned a side gig into a full-time gig, and some had been laid off and were trying to make a go of running their own businesses.

A lot of businesses were made that way. Companies still needed the services, but slashing headcounts was also still needed even as the recession slowed, so consulting—executing tasks once done in-house—became a thing. I'm not sure it was the start of the surge in the gig economy, but I suppose it helped, along with the fact that online services like staffing and bookkeeping and business-card-making websites eventually made it super easy to launch and run a small operation on one's own from anywhere—no pricey office rental required.

Either way, there were eight or so of us there to gather and boost each other over eggs and coffee; we called our meetings the Break Free Club.

I hadn't exactly broken free. I still had a day job, but my side gig had picked up steam.

When I worked in television, I really loved it, and I thought I was good at what I did. Plus, I had done *only* that for so long that I didn't know if I was good at anything else. When I first got laid off, I was certain I was not. My confidence eroded at a rate I'd never previously experienced. While my initial conclusion was that, as a TV producer, I had no real or tangible skills, I started remembering that big win with *Urban Skinny*.

As a producer, I read the newspaper every morning. I made sure everyone else could do their jobs on a shoot. I wrote copy for the prompter in incomplete sentences…with lots of…for pausing on air…and routinely fit stories into ninety seconds. I lived and died by the clock. I told the truth. I got the facts straight. I could ask a long stream of questions and still find more to ask. I drank with the crew. None of those things seemed like actual professional skills. Outside of work, I was an excellent parallel-parker, derived from seven years living in Hoboken, New Jersey (the Mile-Square City), where I learned to cram my car into the tiniest spot, even if it meant a little bumper-nudging of other cars to make mine fit. I can open a wine bottle with great speed and precision because, during summers at university, I worked in a fancy restaurant in Niagara-on-the-Lake, Ontario, with white linens and expensive food.

I didn't see any of those things as translatable into corporate-America-type jobs, but collaborating on books, that started to seem doable. In fact, that first book led to ghostwriting a second book. And a second led to a third. I was working around the clock, and the potential to ghostwrite self-help books full-time became real.

The Break Free Club would meet once a month to talk through our new roles as freelancers and balance the dream versus the reality of professional life. We'd systematically go around the table and report on the wins, the challenges, and the commitments to ourselves for the month ahead. I liked this process, and it inspired me enough to think I could maybe tackle the writing thing full-time.

Having said that, there was some hocus-pocus involved, philosophically speaking, as our group was led by an aspiring life coach. She told us that the Universe was definitely going to play a role in our breaking free. I liked what this coach had to say. Plus, we were all deeply hoping that this new ability to be free and be our own deciders would allow us to flourish. The life coach had us write checks to ourselves for a million dollars, and once, during a weekend meeting, we spent a full afternoon making vision boards.

This vision board was a *real* vision board, much more upscale and specific, with cut-out words too, like an old-school ransom note. My dreams were taped to colorful construction paper, which probably increased their odds over that old magnetic board in Harlem.

I started to believe.

Looking back now though, I'd like to poll the most successful people in the world and find out if they had vision boards.

Hey, Barack Obama: Did you have a vision board?

What about you, Lady Gaga?

Serena Williams—did you cut out a silver Wimbledon tray and tape it to your wall, or did you go out and practice your sport and put in the hard work needed to be a champion?

I suppose I could have continued to put in hard work both working in the news by day and writing books by night, but instead I cut out pictures and taped them to construction paper. And then I stared at it. For some reason, that made more sense at the time than, say, going back to school or networking. Or writing more.

Plus, at these meetings, there was a constant drumbeat of "Don't return to a job...it will hamper your ability to build a business." The prevailing wisdom was to hold out *at any cost* to preserve the time to make your writing or design or filmmaking business work. To an extent, I understood this notion. The words resonated while, at the same time, they tugged at the practical side of my brain.

I didn't want to short myself and miss out on that damn potential I wasn't living up to, but I also wanted to pay my bills *at any cost* first.

There was also a slight undercurrent—when we talked about what we did to earn money that wasn't exactly in line with the mission of breaking free and doing what we loved—we needed to apologize for, or at least rationalize, why we did it. There was a theory that all work had to feed your soul. But some work simply had to feed my mortgage.

This noise eventually put me at a professional crossroads. Though nothing in my life to that point had led me to believe I was an entrepreneur, I was disillusioned with what had become of the news business, or at least what it had become for me. I wasn't working anywhere near where I wanted to. I was still broken from the trauma of getting laid off, and as I tried to look ahead at my prospects, they didn't feel so bright. But I had worked so insanely hard to find another job, the thought of quitting to start a business seemed downright *moronic*. Still, as the self-help ghostwriting work trickled in, so did the thoughts of spending more time on that line of work.

The Grappa Epiphany

Two years after I was laid off, I was sitting at the bar in a restaurant where my neighbor Doug and I used to meet weekly. It was a full hundred blocks from our Harlem apartments. We jokingly called it our local hangout, as we both dreamed of living much further downtown than we were, though I doubt Doug had a vision board anywhere but in his head. I always ordered the exact same thing: an endive salad and the Bolognese pasta

(I like what I like). And I had a crush on the bartender, Tommy (I like what I like). As such, Tommy would often convince me to buy a more expensive wine than I should have.

One night while waiting for Doug (and drooling over Tommy), I mulled over the horror show that had become my day job and how I could build a business on my own and control my own destiny, rather than wait for someone in some office somewhere to crunch some numbers and lay me off again. Plus, I had been watching the show *House of Lies*, about a consulting firm, so while I didn't have an MBA to guide me as I attempted to run a business, I felt I had learned a lot about billing and such, though in a less ruthless and racy manner than theirs.

Regardless of my inexperience or ability to break free, it was officially, glaringly apparent that my job was not for me, and if I had any potential, I was never going to realize it or live up to it there. So that night, at my wannabe local-local, I found myself staring at a row of grappa bottles up on the wall. I don't even like grappa, but the bottles were fascinating to look at. And there were tons of them—twenty or so—all beautiful odd and varied shapes, glass-and-clear-liquid art. I was mesmerized by how pretty they were, wondering how many varieties of grappa there could be and whether they all tasted the same amount of gross. As I pondered them, I had a strange and unfamiliar feeling of confidence wash over me.

Lost in thought, I metaphorically stumbled across a message in the bottle. Well, one in the form of a wall of grappa.

It read: *Bet on you.*

Bet on you.

The Universe was speaking. Or was it my long-lost confidence?

Either way, it was strangely loud, and it formulated rather quickly in my brain. Was I going to continue to work at what felt like a dead-end job? Was the anxiety of living on high alert, wondering when the hammer would next come down on my fate at the hands of another human resources person, worth it? We hadn't come out of the recession fully. Jobs and projects were still going away. Things did not feel secure.

Betting on myself meant taking my fate into my own hands. Jump, and all the stuff on my new and improved vision board would form.

Would it, though?

Writing other people's books had potential, but it was uncertain. But my job was, too. Somewhere in my logic, I considered that, if a single woman with only one mouth to feed couldn't do it, who could? Strangely, at a time when my confidence tank was depleted and fueling me with only fumes, I had the conviction buried somewhere inside to quit and start my own business.

Sitting by and letting someone else drive was, apparently, not my thing. Reflecting on the machine inside me that turned on when I needed to find a job, I realized that I was a survivor. I was never going down with the ship. If I had learned one thing about myself, that was it.

When I was deep in it, sadly, my job loss seemed like a weakness, and my inability to find a job an indication of my shortcomings. It was only later that I realized all of that was just what was inside my head. Certainly, those thoughts wouldn't have crossed my mind when witnessing anybody else struggling to find a job.

But, hey, not many of us offer ourselves the same level of dignity and respect we give to others. (I later read that in a self-help book.)

Friends later commented on how impressed they were that I'd tackled that job search like I had, and in a way that they said they would never have been able to. Thinking about those comments, in that moment—both the insanity of it all and the motivation—I decided that I had the strength to cut my losses, and my 401k (gulp), and jump ship to go it alone.

Maybe ego was involved to a certain degree. Maybe I wanted to leave on my own terms. Maybe I could not face being shown the door. Choice is, after all, choice. Maybe being laid off a second time, which was entirely possible, was not how I wanted my story to go. So I rewrote it.

There I was, just two years after a herculean effort to find a job, and I was quitting one. Bold move? Yes. Brave or stupid? Hard to say. Probably both. But once the decision was made, and my parents hesitantly got on board (at least they said they were, but only after telling me that Uncle Burt said it was nearly impossible to make a living as a writer), I did it. Considering the agony of the previous two years and the number of people I knew who had lost work and never quite landed it again, it was a perplexing and audacious move, and I'm sure, to many who had watched me buckle under the pressure of the job search, completely idiotic. But it suddenly felt right—like, the rightest thing. I felt oddly calm in a way I had not previously.

At the very least, I would be in charge of my destiny. No boss or corporation would be the decider in my career. Stephanie, Inc. would call the shots and, as such, I felt confident I would survive. I had learned that much. I was taking my professional destiny into my own hands. As crazy as it was, I knew in my gut it was the right move.

Plus, I had that million-dollar check pinned to my wall, so I was probably going to be good.

Self-Help: Occupational Hazard or Personality Disorder?

Jumping off a cliff and starting my own business writing self-help books for well-known experts meant that it wasn't just the vision board that got me hooked on finding the fix to all the holes that surely must have existed in my mind, body, and soul. Being obsessed with personal growth and self-help, in fairness, suddenly became my full-time job.

Writing a book *for* someone is actually writing a book *with* them. Twenty or more hours of their time is required just to get started— mostly with interviews and talking through their life or their life's work. It's intimate in a sense, because they have to open up and trust me with their life story or body of work, their insecurities, and the stories they aren't certain they want to share.

It gets personal.

An interviewer by trade, I love asking questions. I pride myself on pulling stuff out of them that maybe they didn't think was important. I often try to make idle chit-chat about seemingly unimportant things, or talk a bit about myself, to spark a conversation unrelated to the specifics of their book. That's when I can hear how a person talks, their voice, and usually learn more about them than I do when they focus on the topic at hand. In those instances, sometimes, the best stuff comes out—

the stuff they wouldn't have thought important. Sometimes it's challenging to figure out how to best demonstrate a protocol they may advise in their book, to get it on the page in a way that the masses may best understand. Talking things through helps.

Generally, whenever someone meets with me to write a book, they will tell me the concept of their book in relation to a previous bestseller. The Marie Kondo of love or the Suze Orman of career coaches; the #GirlBoss of whatever or the Phil Knight of blah-blah. In fairness, there is something to be said for banking on previous winners; we see it in movies all the time.

For me, that means a lot of reading and research before I embark on someone's diet book or career book. If an expert I'm working with offered up a diet plan, I'd do it, measuring food, eating at certain times, and analyzing how I felt along the way. I try to understand how it made me feel, whether something was confusing or simple, so I could best explain it to the reader.

One book I worked on asked the reader to make some consumption adjustments, but also to do some tests, including sending in a hair sample to check for heavy metal toxicity in their body. I figured I would try it to really get to the heart of the book and figure out what the author was trying to accomplish. I clipped a small chunk of hair and sent it to California. A note came back saying I hadn't cut the hair properly, hadn't supplied enough; I had done it wrong. So, I cut another larger chunk from the back of my head and sent that in. The results came back, and some numbers were high according to the chart and some were low, but honestly, I didn't have a clue what they meant or how to interpret them, so I did nothing.

Later, while I was having my hair blown out, the stylist put the hair dryer down, got serious, and said, "You don't have to tell me,

ZEN BENDER

•

50

but I want to let you know you're in a safe space if you choose to. You have a very large chunk of hair cut from the back of your head. Is your partner abusing you? Cutting your hair to demonstrate his power?"

I thanked her for her concern and explained it was a self-inflicted hack job, executed all in a day's work.

Writing books is enlightening, and I'm always learning something new. Twenty or more books into this second career, after discussing sex tapes and drug sprees (my clients', not my own), I had to write something for a scientist who studies sex as medicine. The first time I met with her at her corporate-looking office, I was clearing some space for my computer and moving a few things around on a desk, including some gadgets with wires coming out of them and clips attached. I mindlessly shuffled stuff around and then I froze.

"Um, what are those things I just moved?" I asked.

"Anal and vaginal probes," she said casually.

"Clean, I hope?" I asked as nonchalantly as I could.

"Sterilized."

I'd never worked with a matter-of-fact scientist before. It was already shaping up to be one of my stranger, though more fascinating, book experiences.

As we worked that day, we spent a lot of time going back and forth on how to practically apply some of her notions. It was challenging. Most protocols, for lack of a better explanation, could be handled on one's own, shall we say. But there was one specific concept that required genital stroking by a partner in order to work properly.

Having written many proposals previously, I knew this question would be raised by potential publishers.

Up next on things you don't expect to be debating during work hours when you wake up that morning:

Me: "So, what about single people? We need an explanation for them in this section. Who will stroke their genitals?"

Doc: "It doesn't have to be a romantic partner; they can get a friend to do it."

Me: "Um. I honestly don't think that's a good option. There's got to be a solo way to handle this."

Doc: "There isn't. They can just call a friend to come over and follow the protocol."

Me: "There's literally nobody I would ever call to come to my home in a pinch to stroke my genitals."

Doc: "I could actually think of at least two people who would help me with this."

Me: "I can actually think of a dozen single friends living in NYC who, like me, would not phone a friend to work over their private parts as a favor."

The doctor did eventually explain an excellent and viable solution we could write about and made the point that there were legitimate organizations that would help address the issue of not having a stroker, as well as a way of making single people not feel weird.

When I take on a client with a self-help, health, or wellness premise, I practice the author's diet plan or their personal improvement regimen. I really live it, so I can assess it. If it's a workout or journal ritual as they would prescribe it, then my experience with it helps me explain the hiccups experienced along the way. (NB: I did not take this approach with the aforementioned sex book, meaning no probes were inserted in my person for the making of that proposal.) Instead, I asked single people I knew who they would call to stroke their genitals. Nobody. Even a coupled-up friend was clear: "I don't think I'd even ask my boyfriend to stroke my genitals for science."

The sex book was the anomaly. The rest, I lived. Simply put: The more books I wrote, the more books I fully experienced. I lived them all. Deeply. Occupational hazard: The more books I wrote about fixes, the more and more holes in myself I found that needed plugging.

As I started a new career, I began growing increasingly susceptible to the fix-me brigade. Life in general, plus all the entirely different set of anxieties that come from working for oneself, made me vulnerable. My self-employed friends and I refer to those stresses as "freelancer's syndrome"—a constant state of heightened anxiety, based on the misplaced certainty that nobody will ever contract you again and that you will starve to death while living in a box on a street corner.

Still, betting on myself gave me more power to avoid living in that box. People who got laid off in 2008 got laid off again and again in the wake of that economy.

Later, as I was writing this book, I asked one of the authors I worked with—also one of my favorite humans—Dr. Ramani Durvasula, why we flock to the fixes and the books. She said there are multiple reasons. We don't like uncertainty, so we call upon psychics to give us some answers. And when we go through struggles, we want to know we're not alone. If there's a self-help book out there offering to fix an ailment, that means perhaps

100,000 other people are feeling what you're feeling. Therefore, those books got popular because they provided a collective belonging we all crave.

That resonated with me. I was never a fan of the unknown, and it was true, as I wrote and as I read, it was nice to know that what bothered or challenged me challenged a lot of other people too. And that it was all okay to discuss, or even ponder.

It was suddenly my job to live self-help. Upgrades, classes, coaches, books—tax-deductible research! A new mission emerged in my life—learn it all and then fix it all. Halfway, or moderate, is not a speed on my gearshift. I was getting paid *and* I was basically getting boatloads of free advice.

But my need for a stronger self-help high eventually ballooned beyond the one-dimensional pictures of a vision board or the words of my clients. So began an insatiable craving for multiple fixes, such as juice-fast retreats, coaches of all kinds, full weeks spent Marie Kondoing my house, journaling protocols, psychics, workshops, and a range of books. The world was force-feeding me spiritual seminars, specialists, and life-altering reads, and I grabbed at them all, hoping for, well, some monumental change that would make me better in every way humanly possible. It was coming at me hard. And all the fixes offered up were incredibly radical, too. No small steps; instead, massive overhauls were promised with a few weeks of effort. They wouldn't be pushing these major remedies if I didn't need them or if they didn't work, right? That's what I told myself.

Voilà—a career based on self-help was born.

And so was my new habit.

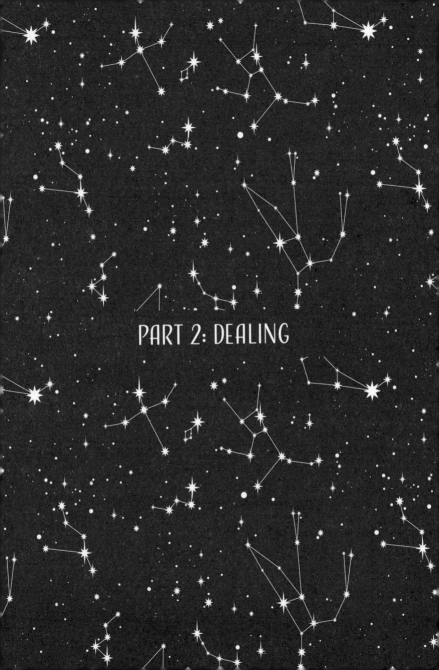

PART 2: DEALING

FAT WOMEN DON'T GET FRENCHED

dating

By the time I reached my forties, it became painfully clear that dating had become like shopping at Marshalls or TJ Maxx. Everything was picked over. The inventory was low and discounted for a reason. All that was left on the shelves were the seconds—damaged, flawed, and ill-fitting. The stuff on the racks was there mostly because nobody else wanted it. At first glance, it was hard to tell what, exactly, was wrong with the goods, but there was always something. (And I'd find it eventually.) Still, I'd try it on anyway, hopeful. Sometimes I would even buy something just to buy something. It wasn't exactly what I was looking for, but it was there, so I grabbed it while I could.

Like discount shopping, dating in my forties meant grabbing the most passable thing I could find because one can't leave empty-handed, but by the time I got home, exhausted from scouring the discount racks for something I didn't even really love, pretending it would work, I was always left with nothing but regrets. Sure, I'd use it once or twice, hoping it would eventually fit, or look better than I expected. But each time, I learned it was never going to change. Frequently, it just came up short and I eventually discarded or donated it, disappointed yet again.

When I was in my twenties, trying to find a partner felt easier, not that I landed one. Dating in your twenties is more like going through the racks at Bergdorf or Saks. The available inventory is generally high-quality, and there's so much more of it—lots of styles, sizes, and colors. You can take your time and look through the racks, try on ridiculous things for fun or things that you know will be great, and consider some wackier ones that you're not sure about. You can splurge and buy something crazy without worrying about the long-term ramifications of having spent your money on a feather-trimmed go-go bolero jacket and having none left for practical black work pants that will last you a decade.

When you are young, you might even be brave enough to buy something you can't quite afford, but that dazzles you, then wear it once and return it with the tags still intact. And if you're broke, you can still window-shop and never actually commit to a single item. There's joy in that.

I dated like that when I was young, but what I didn't realize was that I wouldn't always have the luxury of making foolish or frivolous purchases. Time runs out on that eventually.

When you're in your thirties, you are more likely searching (somewhat frantically) for the father of your child, and maybe feeling somewhat desperate about it. The pressure is really on. The clock is ticking. The inventory is shrinking. Judgment is clouded.

For me, dating in my thirties looked like that episode of *Laverne & Shirley* when they won a shopping spree at a grocery store. They were on the clock, and whatever groceries they could get across the line before time ran out, they got to keep. (As a kid I watched this episode with my dad, and he told me if I ever won a shopping spree just to grab all the steak because it's the most expensive item in the store. #LifeLesson #HoldingOutHopeToWinAShoppingSpree.)

Laverne and Shirley overloaded their cart, stuffed items down their pants, and ultimately couldn't carry everything they had hopelessly grabbed, let alone walk to the finish line, so by the time they dragged themselves to the end, the only items they got to keep were fish sticks and scooter pies. Junk. Limited value added.

They wanted too much, shot too high. They had big expectations and, in the end, got next to nothing.

Restocking the Dating Shelf

A couple of years into my new career as a ghostwriter, I started to get my professional stride. In the career category, early signs indicated that the Universe had been onto something.

There was a steady-ish stream of work coming in, and while I never exactly became a calm and relaxed person in terms of worrying about paying the bills, I had enough work coming in to keep me going. That meant I spent 100 percent of my time focusing on building that business. Losing a job, freaking out about it non-stop, and making radical career choices based on the Universe allowed for little else. That was all the capacity I had at the time.

I was no longer the multi-tasking producer I once had been. Sectioning my life into separate entities was suddenly how I began to get by. That meant, since business was going okay and I was gaining momentum working for myself, it was probably time to start to pay attention to some other aspects of my life.

Dating seemed the obvious aspect to tackle first. That's what all the books said, anyway.

One book I was working on chronicled the dating disasters of a celebrity and all her friends. I was interviewing a long list of women about their dating calamities. One of my favorite stories involved a woman crawling out the bathroom window at a restaurant to escape a horrible first date. These women, all of them, went on tons and tons of dates—they were playing the volume game. By sheer odds alone, it felt like each one of them would eventually meet someone because they were putting effort into it. I found myself cheering them on as I wrote their stories, thinking each time they were getting closer to finding a match.

That inspired me. And since I had made it a habit to put into practice whatever book I was writing, I at least had to try to get back out there.

Like any decent self-help convert, I assessed both the holes in my own life and the available and appropriate experts to help me fix them.

Shopping analogies aside, my first consideration as I developed a strategy was taking an honest account of my dating life. I could sum it up simply by saying: Nobody had really been all that interested. Not for the long haul anyway.

Period.

But that would make for a boring and short chapter and would also not leave much room for self-reflection.

Also, I was working from home, so not only did I not have access to people "at work," I had substantially less interaction with humans in general. (Ask anybody who works from home: It's a lot of alone time.) I needed inventory.

And I had to widen my pool—laws of attraction and all that aside, this was also a numbers game. And in fairness, statistically, the numbers weren't exactly on my side. One stat I found said that there were, apparently, eighty-six single men for every hundred single women. Another—thirty-three available men for every fifty women.

Those numbers rang particularly true in New York. Cities like Portland and Seattle, from what I read, seemed to have better odds, but before I moved across the country seeking Mr. Right, I was certain I could find simpler ways to beat them.

Factoring in age, those numbers were probably worse. The inventory was obviously better when I was younger. But my methodology for finding a single man, any single man, was going to be harder. I went on blinders (my word for a blind date) back in the day. Back in my twenties, my friends had people to set me up with. And there were some good dates that maybe I should have given more consideration. At the time, though, I was often sent away on an assignment and I ended up brushing off many of those good ones.

Ultimately, my friends ran out of options, or more likely hope—I am not sure which one. Either way, I could no longer count on that method to boost my dating inventory and my odds.

Choosing to ease my anxiety, I swore off speed dating. It was efficient, sure. But I had endured the humiliation of it too many times to give it another chance. If you haven't done it, picture this: The women in attendance took a seat at a restaurant—either at various separate tables, or in one instance a U-shaped bar with upholstered benches hugging the wall. We remained stationary while the guys circulated through. Depending on the set-up, I would experience between ten and *thirty* "dates" lasting between three and five minutes each. It was exhausting, torturous, and beauty-pageant-esque.

Kill me. Please.

To round out my plan, I had to be honest with myself about my abilities. One final consideration as I planned to embark upon my dating mission: a quick self-assessment made me start to suspect that I had limited skills, making the shopping that much more challenging. I read the hit book *The Rules* way back when it came out, but I'd also fully ignored all the rules they offered up. For example, if you called me on a Thursday back then (or now) for a date on a Friday, I'd break the not-past-Wednesday thing and say yes.

Read: *Desperate.* Why? Because I dated by employing the same tenacious techniques that I had as a journalist.

Unrelenting.

Make it happen.

Pin it down.

Hot pursuit.

Get the interview at all cost.

Call until the source says yes.

In the words of Meredith Grey, I was more of a "Pick Me, Choose Me, Love Me" type. Iron grip.

In retrospect, that may have scared men off.

For example, for a brief time while I was working for CNBC, I lived in London. On one trip back from New York, I was seated on what was then a Continental Airlines flight, deep in the heart of coach. The flight had just taken off and gotten to cruising altitude, and I had reclined my seat. Within seconds, the woman behind me (British and a tad weathered-looking) started slamming the back of my seat, calling me a fucking bitch over and over, hitting the seat so violently, I was bouncing back and forth like a slow-moving game of paddleball.

She caused such a stir that the flight attendants came by to investigate what was happening. I was a little shell-shocked, frankly. I moved my seat forward into the fully upright position to calm the conflict, but that didn't help. She kept kicking and pushing, screaming obscenities. It became clear that she had hit the bottle before boarding and wasn't just angry at my seat reclining, but basically at everything.

I have flown hundreds of thousands of miles. This had never happened before, and it has never happened since. This was the year 2000, by the way, so for what it's worth; September 11 hadn't yet occurred, and bad behavior on airplanes was perhaps tolerated. I'm not sure Crazy Crammed Weathered Lady's actions would have warranted the plane turning around and landing, but she might have had her wrists put into plastic shackles or been spoken to by an air marshal, at the very least.

Fortunately, the flight attendants just moved me. All of economy was sold out, but there was one empty seat in the front of the plane. That also wouldn't happen today, with computerized upgrades for frequent fliers and all of that. Still, pre-innovation, seat 7L was mine.

The seat was not the only lucky part of this. Beside me was a scruffy and rumpled but super cute young guy with messy light brown hair, who worked in banking in London. Uh, this was the Universe, pre-me-knowing-what-the-Universe-was, putting me in the right place for a reason. I learned through conversation (or a journalistic grilling) that this interesting guy I was suddenly seated next to had been to a conference in Las Vegas.

During my conversation, err…interrogation, I was able to get from him the name of the conference, the name of the hotel he'd stayed at, and the name of the bank he worked for, but not his last name. We had a great talk, and one of us had a car waiting at the airport in London, which we shared into the city. I don't remember whose company paid for the car, but I got out first at my flat in Chelsea. I recall that much.

The next day at work, I shared the details of my plane adventure and meeting of aforementioned cute banking guy with a colleague or two. The consensus following our top-level confab regarding my trans-Atlantic plane experience was that I needed to track him down.

To say that I love a good challenge is putting it mildly.

I immediately got down to business, sort of the way I might have tried to line up interview subjects for a story. Armed with limited information and my ability to impersonate a personal assistant, I called the hotel in Vegas and (believe it or not) successfully got a last name. Then, by calling the bank's main number, I got their standard email address (first-name-dot-last-name@bankname. com)—bingo, I had this guy's email. I am not sure that would happen today (pretty sure it would not) either. But I was impressed with my ~~stalker~~ keen detective skills then and frankly still am to this day.

I sent him a simple note. Subject: *Drink?* Body of email: *Stephanie, Seat 7L.*

His response: *Sure.*

Holy shit! It had worked.

We made a plan. At the time, it didn't really strike me that my behavior was offensively aggressive. When we finally did get together, it became clear it had freaked him out and that he was only there to find out how I had tracked him down. Unfortunately, the entire conversation focused on that topic. Clearly, one of us was a better detective.

I didn't tell him anything, just laughed at each inquiry like a dumb girl (though damn I would have liked to have shared my brilliant tactics), but his assumption was that I was part of the "American Mafia" (he said that with a straight face, like he believed it) or that I'd gone to the trouble of hiring a detective. (Uh, I was hard up, but not desperate. Not quite.)

Okay, so looking back, that sort of assertive behavior might be exceptional for chasing news stories, but also might be frowned upon, invasive, and a little cuckoo-slash-I'm-not-going-to-be-ignored-Dan *Fatal Attraction*-esque when chasing guys.

So that was that. He never called. Scared of me having a hit put out on him by Uncle Sal, or just disinterested, I'll never know.

In fairness, the Universe had teed me up. It gave me the potential to find a partner. Having said that, there was some operator error wiping out the Universe's good work.

Shiny Hair, Shiny Ovaries

Looking back on that London episode as a standard measure and perfect articulation of my Meadow Soprano-esque dating skills, I knew that eventually I would have to call in the professionals to help me develop a multi-pronged approach to finding a date so that, if the Universe provided for me once again, I wouldn't muck it up. I'd be *more ready*.

My first stop was enrolling in a seminar aptly offering a lesson in why I must suck at dating, titled *Why You're Single*. There was a promise in the literature, but I can't remember what it was. Obviously fixing the being-single part of one's life was the main nugget.

My friend Sarah and I went together. We were both hopeful that we would learn something about ourselves and the skills needed to find a husband before our eggs dried up for good, but as we entered a banquet-type room at a hotel in New York, looking around at all the hopeful and yet equally slightly embarrassed-to-be-there women, we grew skeptical.

There were hundreds of women eager to fix the flaw of not yet having found a mate. It was a sea of sad-sack singles. Surely

Sarah and I were better than this. That was my first thought. My second was: *This is going to be a waste of my time.*

The woman leading the seminar opened by saying that, if we were showing up with the attitude that we knew better and that this seminar was dumb, but we grudgingly came with a friend, then we were not going to learn anything.

Hmm. Okay, so she was a mind reader.

I made my best *I'm listening* face and tried to control the number of times I rolled my eyes.

Initially, two things struck me as semi-interesting. First, she explained that men sometimes want to get our attention by giving us a gift. That lets us know they have noticed us and lets them snoop around a bit to see if we have noticed them too, or if they could inspire us to notice them with a tiny gesture. For example, the teacher said, should a guy at work drop off a pen at your desk just because he had been to the supply closet, accept it. That's a gift. Don't say, "I don't need a pen."

Like I probably would have or had often done.

And then, be open-minded. Maybe the pen giver wasn't on your radar, but maybe he should be.

Both seemed to me like sound pieces of advice. Later, the former transcended dating for me. I started to try to be gracious when anybody did something small but nice for me, or accept what they offered up for whatever reason, because perhaps that was what they had to give. Over time, I started to notice more closely the tiny gestures that people made and to receive them all with the same amount of gratitude. Perhaps it made them feel good to do a little something for someone else, and perhaps saying thanks and accepting a gesture was just the right thing to do.

My attitude, as I sat in my seminar, slightly adjusted. Not fully, but slightly.

But then she lost me.

Her next piece of advice: Keep your hair shiny. Why? If you have shiny hair, a man will definitely think you're fertile, and subconsciously think you are wife material.

Think about that.

The only way to land a husband was to demonstrate that my ovaries were pumping out prime grade-A eggs, and the only way to do that was with long shiny hair.

News flash: My hair *was* shiny. My hair had always been shiny.

As I sat there and listened, I was suddenly horrified. As a feminist. As a human. As a person who hoped there were better ways to demonstrate that you had the potential to be a solid life partner.

As someone with shiny hair.

Itching for an opening, Sarah and I could not wait to bolt.

Once class broke for coffee, I left that seminar. Sadly, it never left me.

As insane as that advice was, as the years marched on and the dating got harder, often all I could think of was…hmm…does he think I'm fertile enough to date? It had snuck into that inner voice in my head and swirled around with all the other nuggets of self-doubt.

And I had let it.

Prospecting in Heels

The seminar an epic fail, I moved on to a book called *Calling in the One*, which basically *guaranteed* you'd find love in seven weeks if you followed the steps strictly. In fact, I had spoken to several people who knew someone who had fallen in love after reading it. Or, in one case, I knew a person who completed the book, and then quickly and unexpectedly found her life partner and married him!

It worked! There was indisputable scientific evidence in front of my face.

At first, I tackled the book hardcore, doing the exercises suggested, one chapter at a time, and being very open-minded to the main takeaway, which frankly was excellent advice: Don't look for the person you have in your mind as your type. Open your eyes and consider other possibilities. We all have preconceived notions of what is or isn't husband material (they don't have to have shiny hair, or hair at all, apparently), and those notions prevent us from opening our eyes to a diamond in the rough that would make a great match. As directed, I also left room for a life partner, making sure, for example, that there was a nightstand on each side of my bed, so the imaginary *he* had one too.

The book was a seven-week sentence. I made it to week five.

Another hurdle: aside from getting bored, I simply didn't have the inventory needed to get me to the finish line. I realized that I could make my hair shine like the bloody sun in July, and I could open my mind, but first, I needed the actual men to at least consider not overlooking.

I was bemoaning my experience to Lara, an editor (and friend), while I was working with her on someone else's book. She gave me a suggestion. She was working with the author of another book—a dating coach—who had published a couple of books on dating. She told me I should investigate, that the advice was extremely helpful.

Instead of just buying the books, I opted to up my game and to outright hire the aforementioned dating coach to get private tutoring. After an initial phone consultation, I dove in, buying the full six-hour session pack, including online-dating-profile-making, phone sessions, and email sessions. It was a lot of money, but it seemed like it would be a worthwhile endeavor because it would help solve my inventory issue by getting me out there and online.

It was immediately clear that the dating coach had a close-the-deal mentality, one that she had applied to finding her own husband after years of working in sales. She applied the salesperson skills to her dating-coach business. She was clear at the onset of our discussion: I was to make dating like making a business deal (okay, so sales skills apply to dating, but journalism skills don't).

No shiny-hair mandate, either.

First, I had to create a profile and get online. I'd done some Match.com decades earlier, when AOL dial-up was a thing, but I hadn't re-entered that murky pool of online shopping after it proved unfruitful.

Her rules for that were quite simple and made sense: Only do the dating platforms that cost money (online dating hadn't become as fully app-driven at that time) because that meant you were pursuing dates that were investing in this process, a.k.a. looking for a relationship, not a fling.

For my profile, I was told to use photos that were full-length, meaning not just head and shoulders, but head to toe.

Gasp a thousand gasps.

I was horrified, but it made sense. You were making clear what inventory you were offering.

Panicked at first, I did what she said. Have the photographer shoot from up high on a ladder because that would take off the extra pounds and eliminate the double chin. Wear bright lipstick, get pops of color into the frame, and always—and this is the not-so-feminist thing—wear a dress and heels in the photo (and when going out on dates…ugh). The touch-ups were to be limited, too, as in—leave my crow's feet in place.

My photos were taken as directed and, much to my surprise, they were unquestionably the best photos I had ever had done. And they were the only recent ones that existed of me in heels and a dress, showing all of my curves. Together, the dating coach and I crafted a profile and posted my photos, and I hit the online circuit.

For that, she offered up some basic rules:

When using a dating site as your main man-meeting place, take *all* dates requested. Turn nothing down. By this point in my life, I had become less choosy, so I welcomed this notion. When someone asked what I was looking for in a man, I said, "Someone who has all of his teeth, and showers regularly." (I was choosier than I thought, and ultimately couldn't abide by this turn-nothing-down notion, but I tried to remain more open-minded than I would have been had I not been coached.)

Also, I was told in a coaching session that dates aren't dates, they're meetings, at first. For me, that helped take the pressure off. Plus, in this artificial world of meeting online, it makes sense to adopt this attitude. What can one possibly glean from a few sentences and a professionally taken photo?

Additional rules:

When communicating, treat emails and texts like a salesperson would, by mirroring the tone of the sender. If a suitor writes only two sentences, you respond with only two. Also, mix up the speed with which you respond (to keep him guessing, I presume, and to make clear you aren't sitting by the phone waiting to hear from him—which I was, of course, because I treated the coaching endeavor like a sport), and never respond on a weekend.

Once you've made an interesting connection, get off the platform and start communicating directly. An initial text or two is fine, but stop texting immediately to force a phone call, so you can get a better read on the person.

Take your time and spread out the courting process to best be able to assess whether the guy you're communicating with is indeed a good person.

Keep that first phone call to thirty minutes max (make him want more).

First meeting: Don't have more than one drink, so you can judge his character and make a good choice, and keep it to one hour (make him want more). I was rather ungraceful at this one-hour thing. On one date, I was deep in conversation when I realized it was a couple of minutes beyond the one-hour cutoff. I interrupted him and, in a panic, said, "I gotta go," stood up, and basically Cinderella-at-midnighted my way out of there.

Dating coach results: One guy actually wanted to marry me. Though it wasn't an on-the-knee proposal, he said a couple of times he could see marriage happening between us, and he came to this conclusion just a few dates in. Frankly, I found that a little creepy, given that he didn't really know me, but rather, perhaps, thought I looked good on paper.

I had less than zero interest in him.

I did, however, play out the dating coach's advice, even though I had an inkling early on that it wouldn't work. Like, within the first five minutes of the first meeting.

Still, my coach said to stick to it to see if there was a good guy in there for the long haul and reminded me not to make my choice based on superficial reasons. I did try that. And I was not being superficial in my thinking.

Don't judge me and think that I only wanted to be with unavailable men and all that stuff people say about chronically single people. In the end, the best way to explain this particular misfire was to say that our values and political viewpoints were far from aligned. That made it a certainty it would not have worked, because, for example, he was strongly in favor of teachers carrying guns in schools, and he thought the finest restaurant in New York was a theme restaurant in Times Square where the staff wore costumes.

Other red flags: He had never heard of a place called the West Village, despite having technically grown up in New York City. I'm not a snob. That's not an I'm-so-fancy comment. I come from as humble beginnings as the next guy. But if you live in New York, the most amazing city in the world, rich with restaurants that offer world-class cuisine for anywhere from ten to five hundred dollars, and you're single, which he was, you gotta be curious enough, or even hungry enough, to once venture out to the West Village to see what's on the menu.

Or try a non-costume-wearing-staff restaurant.

I saw it through, though, assessing the experience, just like the dating coach told me to do, until it seemed I had been as open-minded as I humanly could have been.

Then I shot the horse and moved on.

But I will say this: Those rules and directives were easier to follow when there was no immediate spark with someone. While Mr. I-Love-Theme-Restaurants was easy to hang up on, later, when I had a date with someone who seriously piqued my interest, I a) drank too much, b) let the evening drag out on date number one for four hours because it was fun, c) didn't follow the mirror exercise, and d) so on and so on.

That didn't go anywhere.

My dating coach's advice didn't revolve around online dating. She had another system for meeting men as well. It was called prospecting. For several Sundays in a row, I would get up, go to the *Drybar* for a blowout, put on the motherfucking high-heeled boots, and go to a coffee shop in a different neighborhood each week. The task at hand was not to read the paper or stare at a phone—rather, it was to work the room. Every time a seemingly single guy went to the milk-and-sugar station, Stephanie went to the milk-and-sugar station.

Not for the milk.

Not for the sugar.

I went to strike up a conversation.

I capital-D-detested this activity. Actually, to say I detested this task is akin to saying that Canadians occasionally say "sorry." (I have a "sorry" habit. I say it a hundred times a day, even if, or especially if, you knock into me.)

Still, I got it done. Coffee-shop prospecting was a nine-to-noon venture. I'd lunch-counter prospect after that, and then I'd men's-clothing-shop-prospect after that. Why waste a good blowout?

Dates yielded from prospecting: zero.

But! I built up my wilted confidence doing so because, as I started talking to strangers (even while wearing sneakers and a ponytail on non-prospecting days), I noticed something interesting: Human beings, even in New York, talked back. And sometimes they checked out my cleavage. Perhaps that wasn't newly happening, but I started to notice it.

Exhausted just reading about prospecting? I promise you it was beyond exhausting. *Calling in the One* said not to complain about the effort because relationships take work, too. Few truer words were ever spoken. It was all work.

I kept at the online dating thing for a while, as I'm not a quitter. But I reached my breaking point one day while on eHarmony, a site on which you spend hours filling out questionnaires and providing particulars and specifics because they use an algorithm to make the most perfect personal connection a computer can make.

I noticed that, after a few months, the matches were less than perfect and found myself knocking my requirements down considerably to widen my pool.

One day, I was given a peculiar connection to consider.

My match was a subway driver. Photo posted with his profile: in the subway car, driving the train, in uniform, with a subway map in his pocket.

Remember, my dating coach said to only go on the sites that I had to pay for because that meant the guys were making an effort, which indicated a desire for a relationship rather than a fling. Not changing out of one's uniform for one's profile picture didn't feel like an effort.

Yet, I had to blow out my hair and wear high heels.

Also, other than the fact that I frequently took the subway, I strove to see how our profiles matched, but I couldn't. At a quick glance, and after a full forensic investigation, it was clear that we had nothing in common.

Saying all this, of course, makes me sound like a mean girl. I understand that. I struggled with passing on that particular match, as I was told clearly to accept all dates. Remember, I told myself as I stared at the photo, these are *meetings*, not dates. I was scoping out a pool of people I might not have otherwise encountered, giving myself exposure to as many people as possible who wouldn't have waltzed through my living room while I watched TV.

It made sense—that it wasn't a date until there was more of a spark or a decision to reconnect after the initial meeting. Judging someone by their photo isn't the way to find true love. I understood that, and I had found myself previously working to be more open-minded and to take meetings even when, in my gut, I didn't think things would work out. But the subway driver situation nagged at me. Rejecting him on the basis of what he did (if that was what I was doing) tugged at my class sensibilities, because

I didn't want to be a dick. And of course, there were the opinions of all the smug and coupled people who gave me the overused "Who knows, he could be really nice."

I felt discouraged, but I knew I had truly tried. Eventually I came to realize that all that I struggled with, and all the advice of the dating coach and the married friends (who would never, by the way, have taken half the "meetings" I and my single friends endured), was, to a degree, dumb if blindly and universally followed.

As a result, I stopped even telling married or coupled people what I was doing. I focused on the singles, out there in the trenches, doing the same thing.

In doing so, I sought the counsel of my friend Alison, a fellow single-woman-of-a-certain-age. She is a doctor of psychology who had hit the online dating scene in an enviable way. Textbook-hard, with precision; multiple dates on any given day.

She too had found it somewhat of a struggle. Often, she found her meetings intellectually unchallenging. She and I had lengthy discussions about this: Was it okay to want to date someone who was as educated as she was? I had a master's degree, but I wasn't as educated as Alison. She had a PhD. Still, the guilt over being choosy was overwhelming for us both. As in, was it fair to ignore the subway driver?

Her research revealed that, *yes*, we could be choosy. More, we *deserved* to be choosy.

She had consulted an expert of her own, who told her that she'd worked hard to get a PhD and a post-secondary degree could be her line in the sand; that it was okay to seek out a professional partner for herself.

And so she did.

And guess what? Her now-husband, we learned later, had also set a high bar for himself. But, unlike Alison and me, he hadn't even remotely struggled with his decision to check the box on his online dating platform for "graduate degree only." (If you've never experienced the horror of online dating, that is indeed a question—along with preferred height, income, religion, and political views, just like the menu at the local seafood shanty. If only it were as easy to land a husband as it is to land some fried clams.)

More, his decision to do so is what led him to find Alison. His only concern was that he was narrowing his pool. But he had done it in reaction to having dated several women previously that he felt might have a hard time carrying on a high-level conversation at a work event. While Alison and I had been questioning whether our choice to shoot for an *equal* was snobby, her now-husband had not.

There was something else that we decided, too: While the stakes for a younger woman are mostly about aging eggs and faltering ovaries, the stakes for women over forty are quite different when dating. Presumably, we'd all worked hard to survive to that point. I had. As the breadwinner, I had bills to pay, and in the mid-forties, I was hit with the realization that retirement was looming, and that added another layer of financial stress to my situation.

Sure, I didn't have kids to pay for. But I had psychics and Reiki and coaches. And a mortgage. And health care.

When the stats revealed that approximately one-quarter of single women live below the poverty level in retirement, as opposed to just 6 percent of those who are married, the stakes soared. Taking on a partner who couldn't afford the bills was a challenge I was ill-equipped to tackle.

The uncertainty of my financial future, based on my lumpy self-employed income, changed the dating equation by the time I hit forty-five. Sure, *Calling in the One* made a fair point: Look in places you might not have. I did. But financial facts sometimes overpower *love will find a way*. And for that, I wouldn't apologize.

I suspect there will be an argument made here by some who say: Women marry men for money all the time and expect to be taken care of. Great work if you can get it. But it wasn't for me. It was not for the 99 percent of the women with whom I associated. And, on the flip side, I know many women who are the breadwinners in their coupled lives, and for them I'm thrilled.

At the end of the day, lowering the bar (whatever that bar was for me) *just because I was of a certain age* would have been the wrong choice. Not only did Alison and I deliberate about wanting an intellectual equal, I recall a time when someone told me to "dumb it down" on a blind date and not to mention that I owned an apartment and a rental property because that was intimidating.

We can all play that very anti-feminist game of letting him do the asking, letting him set the tone of the conversation, and letting him drive the pacing of the relationship, but I suspect that's setting the table for the relationship as well. I'm unapologetically opinionated. I'm unapologetically smart. Settling was not the way to go; rather, waiting for that great value-added guy out of *want*, not *need*, is quite okay by me.

All of this is not to say that I won't meet a great guy who I wouldn't have expected to be a match. But when I was filling out forms, checking boxes, and being ruthlessly judged both by the men reading my profile (I assume, based on the low volume of interest) and by the friends who accused me of being choosy and suggested that I settle when my gut was telling me not to, then the criteria, to me, are very different. Being unapologetically choosy simply seemed part of the equation—baked in from the start because of the questionnaire—rather than simply meeting someone, liking him, and worrying about the details later. Match services feature unnatural, built-in judgment, forced choices, and checklists.

And maybe the subway driver was conducting some sort of experiment and was really a nuclear physicist but wanted to see who wasn't too shallow to consider him, but I wasn't ready to find out.

And with that last match, I deleted my profile and took a break from online dating.

The Modern-Day Spinster

I like to learn from any situation—my mistakes, my wins, and my awkward encounters. Dating and all my classes and experts and quests included. For a long time, I felt stressed about my non-marital non-status, which was in part why I worked so hard to fix it. I thought it said something negative about me, that there must be something seriously wrong with my character. In fairness, I also did it because the company and grounding of a life partner would be nice.

As I thought about the work I'd put in, I also gave some thought to society's and the world's opinion of being single and how that may have clouded my judgment and pushed me to actually worry about how shiny my hair was.

Single men are bachelors. Single women are spinsters. Spinster, in the world's eyes, is not a good look.

The definition of an Old Maid: *A single woman regarded as too old for marriage.* A bachelor, on the other hand, is viewed as virile and young. Probably with shiny hair, too. There's no equivalent.

That makes me and a long list of friends *un-marry-able.* Old Maid, childless spinster pals, who are way past our prime.

That notion has certainly been reinforced by society. I remember shortly after first moving to Hoboken, after graduate school, I'd return to my hometown and see people who I had worked summer jobs with or people from high school. The conversation would often go something like this:

Random judgy person: Hey, Stephanie, what have you been up to?

Me: Hey, I got my master's degree at Syracuse (and a scholarship when I got there!), and then I got a job in TV in New York!

Random judgy person: But have you met anybody?

Me: No, not yet. But I bought my own apartment (before turning thirty) and I have covered the Olympics (in Australia) and interviewed tons of celebrities, and even Fidel Castro, and I lived in London for a year while working for the network (acting bureau chief!), traveled all over the world (etc. etc. etc. etc. etc. etc. etc. etc.).

Random judgy person: But still single? That's too bad.

Rinse and repeat.

That was standard-issue return-to-hometown conversation. It got stale after a while. It still happens on occasion, and it's still stale. Or else—as most of my single-at-this-age friends agree—everybody just thinks you're a lesbian, but too afraid to come out.

One day, when I was doing research for someone's book, I needed to find out about the purchasing power of single women over forty. I learned that if I typed in *single wo*… all I got was a stream of stories intended to help single women get over a common ailment: being single.

10 Reasons Single Women Over 40 Make Amazing Dates

If You're Single Over 40, Should You Ever Settle?

2 Huge Reasons Single Women Over 40 Have a Hard Time Finding a Partner (Answer: you're too picky)

What Does a Single Women in her 40s Do with Her Life?

The 5 Types of Single Women in Their 40s

In case you're interested in learning what I was actually looking for: Single women account for more real-estate purchases than single men according to the National Association of Realtors. Despite lagging incomes, our spending clout is significant (the She Economy is, apparently, a thing). Single adults now outnumber married ones, and a 2014 stat showed that 62 percent of the adult population has *never* been married, double the percentage in 1960. Single women are now a powerful voting block too. The Census Bureau recently revealed there are more single fifty-something women in the United States than ever before.

When many people think about single women over forty, they often think how sad it is for them to be single, like it's an illness.

Given all the heroic measures I had gone to in order to change my circumstance, it became clear that I thought of myself that way, too.

Bottom line: It's hard to feel comfortable with a life ~~circumstance~~ choice when nobody else does.

It's hard to differentiate between what's right for your life and what you think is right for your life, based on what everyone else dumps on you as a measure of success in life.

It made me wonder: Shouldn't we older single women be harnessing that power to do something other than compromise and apologize?

I use highbrow terminology for that: People dump their shit on you. All. Day. Long. Not just dating stuff either. Their insecurities with their lives and their successes. Their *need* for, rather than *want* for, a relationship.

And I say all of this fully admitting I was (am) looking for, but not finding, that guy to be my life partner. But, as I assessed my life to date in reverse order as it pertained to being single, the fact remained that I was presented with an insanely exciting job at a young age, a job that, even looking back now, I would not have traded for anything.

I traveled all over the world chasing newsmakers. Me. Regular young and naive me from St. Catharines, Ontario, Canada. Inexperienced. Hopping on and off planes and checking into fancy international hotels on someone else's dime. That was thrilling—more exciting than the clown I met at speed dating who didn't want to pay for a drink at a bar on our one follow-up date. Instead, he brought little bottles of Sambuca (of all things) and asked if I wanted to take one into the bathroom and pour it in my glass; no (I'm leaving now) and no.

I preferred getting on a plane to Sun Valley, Idaho, to cover the big-thinking Allen & Company Media Conference, or covering a Super Bowl somewhere, or standing in every Major League Baseball dugout at spring training in Florida and interviewing the players for a series on the business of baseball.

Maybe Mr. Sambuca would have been okay. But landing interviews with Jeffrey Bezos or Michael Ovitz or you name it was a lot more exciting. Don't get me wrong: Plenty of busy TV producers manage to meet their eventual life partners while also jetting off to interview luminaries. But I wasn't focused on it. Not my A-focus, anyway. Not while I was in my prime and didn't know that my face would sag and my hair would get gray. My A-focus was on landing a plum assignment. My B-focus was on landing a bruised plum of a date.

I was born in 1969. And I have a lot of friends who are essentially my age who currently have no life partner and some who have never been married. There are some who met their mates deep into their forties but divorced them. Professionally, these single or single-for-a-long-time friends of mine kick serious ass at work. Lawyers, corporate executives, managing directors, fine art brokers—powerhouses, all of them.

Those judgy people who kept asking if I'd met anyone clearly hadn't read or understood *The Feminine Mystique*, the book that called out the false concept that our place, our only place, was in the home as a mother and homemaker. It wasn't. It isn't.

But, I'll admit, we had perhaps experienced a Feminist Mistake— window-shopping, not buying or committing, thinking time was never-ending. (Nobody told me then that eggs get old, the baby oil you used to put on your face to tan at sixteen will show up at forty in the form of spots, and the inventory for finding a life partner will shrink considerably. Well, maybe they did. But I didn't listen.)

Maybe I was five minutes too old to hear about the concept, but I had never met anybody who'd frozen their eggs. I could be wrong, but I feel like my generation of women is maybe the first that, en masse, was able to grab at professional opportunities, and who chose to do so as a priority over finding a partner. Not that we didn't want one, but the doors were kicked open at our jobs and we were proudly storming in with glee.

I will allow myself this: At some point during this dating blitz, I found a little peace with myself. I accepted my starring role in *This Is the Life I Made*, not *These Are the Cards I Was Dealt*, and with the decision to take children off the table (because at some point it gets a bit rusty up there), the faucet was loosened, the pressure was off, and the conscious decision to only let value-added people into my life made dating different. More enjoyable. Once I figured out that I could go to Paris alone if I felt like it and I didn't need a date…the doors opened up.

Do I have dating fatigue? Yes. Over the years, so many people said, "You gotta put yourself out there." I have. I do. I'm tired. I get rejection all day long as a writer, pitching and pitching and pitching. It cuts deep, but not as deeply as dating rejection. That's emotionally exhausting. So is choosing outfits and staying out late and pushing through the painful awkwardness of a first meeting with someone you don't know who has nothing to say. If you've done it, you can relate. If you haven't, trust me when I say, it is a lot.

But the good news is, after trying all the books and the coaches and the online dating, I have at least figured out that the stakes don't feel so high anymore. The tick-tock of the clock is less noisy. All in due time. The only good thing about dating later in life: My thinking started to change for the better. Wisdom and experience began to feed my decisions, not just coaches and books. I started to realize that relationships would not look the way I thought they would look when I was twenty.

And that was okay.

I also learned a few tools from my efforts that I'll employ, and some of the things that just didn't feel right, too (a little anti-feminist to say the least). And, with all the preaching about authenticity, I've fully dismissed any tactics that require any form of dating deception (not that I ever embraced any of it). You get what you pay for in some sense. Friends who have acted breezy and created a persona to land a guy have then had to live with the ramifications of not having a say in the day-to-day once the ploy worked.

We are different people than we were in our twenties and thirties. And, despite the trauma of decades of more bad dates than I care to recall, and the disappointment when one that I kind of liked didn't feel the same, at least in my forties, I was finally experienced enough to know that it would still all be okay. I have built a good life and it will go on.

Plus, there's this thing called hope. And that will eventually get me back in the game.

And because of hope, I will always keep shopping. Even at Marshalls. Because every once in a while, there's an Isabel Marant blazer on the rack that's in perfect condition and fits just right, that I know I'll have and wear forever. Or at least there's the potential that such a unicorn exists.

CHAPTER 5

NUMEROLOGISTS, CLAIRVOYANTS, AND HEALERS, OH MY!

spirituality

Nowhere do enlightenment and bliss feel more achievable and available for purchase than in Venice Beach, California. Nobody there seems to work, so they seemingly have time to fill achieving peace. And everyone, no matter who you talk to, is a believer in the pursuit of healing the mind, body, and soul. They juice, they chant, and they don't make decisions that aren't psychic—or healer—approved. People are painfully familiar with the lunar calendar, the latest New Age remedy, and of course, Mercury in retrograde, which, it seems, is taking place: All. The. Time.

Venice is a place of contrasts too—littered with both young people, lunching and surfing and trotting around on electric scooters (annoying), and the old guard: the real hippies who laid claim to the beach zone decades ago, who have dress flip-flops and casual ones. Both have made Venice a true state of mind, not just a zip code, one that permeates its population's every move and every meal, and can be felt in every item for sale on its boardwalk (and now couture-filled retail zone), Abbott Kinney. It's both frozen in time and a snapshot of progress as seen by the gutter-less, colorful bungalows beside the modern, concrete, steel and glass, high-rise homes that have been squeezed onto a thousand-square-foot lot, thanks to the surge of dotcoms and apps that have infiltrated the vibe.

But that vibe is its allure. When I first started spending time in Venice, I didn't just look around. I inhaled. Deeply.

Guru Ground Zero

The writer's life, like Venice, grew to be a world of contrasts.

I quickly discovered that the freedom of working for oneself was a stress-filled curse rich with an entirely new menu of anxieties, but it was also completely glorious in multiple ways. There was no more Sunday-night angst ahead of Monday-morning blues back at work. There was no more six o'clock scramble to catch the subway to the office. Sure, there were endless hours of time to fill and schedule, but those hours, I learned, could be filled anywhere on earth.

My anywhere became Los Angeles in the winter.

When I first started working for myself, I sponged off my friend Karyn, who generously allowed me to stay with her in LA for long periods of time. She didn't just offer accommodation and good wine, but frequently some words of wisdom as well. Not found in any self-help book, her words kept me going when I thought of quitting (often) and returning to a day job with health insurance, because it might have been easier than slogging away on my own.

Once, when I said as much to Karyn, she offered up some key thinking. She said, and I'm paraphrasing, not to pull the rip cord on my new business until I absolutely had to because, once I did so, I would probably never try to work for myself again.

And so, despite the occasional struggle or speedbump that came my way, I stayed the course. I waited it out, and it eventually paid off. Because, as people struggled with a stalled economy, they increasingly, it seemed, turned to self-help books. Previously in publishing, it seemed like the hot trends were books by Real Housewives and Snooki. And then suddenly there was a flood of diet books and self-help books by experts, many of whom needed help writing them. And that was good for business.

That meant that, eventually, I didn't have to be a sponge, which was good because I hated being a sponge. I was able to rent my own little bungalow in Venice.

Renting in Venice, by the way, was an interesting endeavor, almost like a pyramid scheme that put me squarely at the bottom. I was renting from a woman who was renting the bungalow from another woman, who was renting the bungalow from the owner. Everybody I knew in Venice was doing something similar, hanging on for dear life, keeping their options open as housing prices soared, never willing to walk away from cheap rent in case they needed it back one day.

The first winter I rented a house in Venice I was particularly fogged up in the brain from whatever was happening at the time. Maybe I was feeling anxious or stressed, about what in particular I don't recall, but for a writer on a deadline, it wasn't a good state of being. No work was getting done, just fretting. After talking to some local friends, I was immediately informed that the only way to clear it out was to hit the New Age action hard. I assembled a list of spiritual experts of varying disciplines.

It was time to insert a little church in my life. Venice offered up the religion and congregation I needed.

Like a good New Yorker, I was ready to throw money at it and embrace even the most seemingly far-fetched spiritual activities.

That made great sense to me.

As I started to research what single practice might be most appropriate, I was entranced by them all. There were so many. It became clear that there was no need to pick and choose. Why approach my urge to reduce my anxiety as an either/or situation, when I could do everything that existed to fix my problem?

And, without any hesitation, I decided that more had to be better, so for every suggestion that came my way, a booking soon followed, until I had fully overloaded my days with appointments in order to reduce my anxiety, figuring that where one fix didn't work, another would pick up the slack.

I'd already dabbled in a few things by this point—I had been cleansing, and dieting, and doing multiple self-help-type activities on the East Coast, but this mission was next-level, and more of an out-there and New Age approach to change and enlightenment. More wacky, sure. But the way I saw it, I had six weeks to make it happen, and I was determined to cram. I was going to get fixed, California-style.

I was going to kill it; my quest for enlightenment was a certainty.

Armed with a list that was long and grew longer, I charted out an A-type-personality mind-body-and-soul regimen certain to brush away the cobwebs and, in the process, make my life great. It included numerology, rainbow healing, sound-bath meditation, acupuncture, Thai massage, yoga, astrology, and frankly, whatever else I could get my hands on. I asked everyone I spoke to for a referral. And believe me when I say that everyone had one to give. Simply put, there was a lot of AFOG (another fucking opportunity for growth) in Venice. An endless supply.

There was a constant stream of unsolicited advice, too. Unprovoked, I was told things like: I wore too much black because I hoped it would act as a protective shell.

Or, as I preferred to think of it: Black hid the extra pounds better than white.

Regardless, I welcomed it all, and soaked up all the wisdom I could take in.

My first stop: The Mystic Bookstore. It's on Abbot Kinney Road and is a Mecca for crystals and incense and tie-dye and feathers and beads and books on fixing all kinds of shit about oneself. And, of course, healers—a wall of names, photos, and their specific practices.

Just walking in there made me feel semi-healed, but I knew I'd be more healed once I sat down with the on-call numerologist.

Back in a little dark room, a very serious man asked me my name, birthday, and birthplace, then didn't utter a word for the first ten minutes. This deeply concerned me, as I'd only signed up for thirty minutes for eighty dollars. I couldn't concentrate as I watched him do some fancy calculations, applying numbers to the letters used in the limited information that I'd provided him. It was like trying to beat the parking meter, knowing time was ticking. Panicked, I wondered if I should zip out to the front desk and quickly buy more time, since nothing was immediately happening and the time was dwindling.

Eventually, he spoke.

I learned that I was a strong eight and nine. In the looks department, I've always considered myself no more than a six, so my immediate assumption was that this had to be a good thing. Higher numbers = better?

Not the case in numerology. This wasn't an appearance-based science.

He explained that those two numbers were somewhat bad together; they stifled one another. Eight spoke to my need and ability to run a business and generate money—abundance and my ability to enjoy it. The problem? The other number canceled it all out. The other number, nine, was my need to do good in the world, likely a result of my modest upbringing. Those two numbers were at odds with each other: that I could in fact succeed in business and be rich (my interpretation), but that my parents being frugal (his words, not mine) taught me it was better to be careful with money, so I constantly resisted being rich.

Personally, I have always felt quite open to being rich.

Still, I started to reflect. Could that have been true? A few things came to mind...

My father will, to this day, into his eighties, bend down and pick up a penny. I might not exert myself in such a way even for a quarter. Maybe a dollar. War-time and post-war children, my parents walked ten miles to school, home for lunch, and back again, every day. You know that story.

When I was young, I wanted a pair of Dominion Precision white roller skates with red wheels. My dad bought me a pair. I opened them up, all shiny and white, and slipped them on. They were big, he said, size eight, so I'd grow into them. I never did. To this day, I only take a size seven or seven and a half.

And once, after I'd moved to New York post-college, my father saw how many pairs of shoes I owned. He said he'd worn the same pair of Florsheim Shoes for twenty-five years. I was in my twenties at the time, so I explained of course that my feet were somewhat smaller twenty-five years back. That new shoes over the years were a necessity.

Shoes aside, there's always a used tea bag on the counter at my parents' house because nobody should use a tea bag just once. It can, after all, make a couple of cups.

The worst and best depression-era-thinking memory I have is of my grandfather on my mom's side. That man was a penny-pincher of monumental proportions. One afternoon, way back in the eighties, we were sitting in our kitchen, with its bronzy-brown appliances and dark brown cupboards, at our oval glass table, eating off our white Corelle plates with blue flowers, when my older sister began to drain a can of tuna liquid (oil or water) into the sink. Suddenly, my grandfather, noticing what she was doing, jumped up and screeched. We were all startled. He approached her, making her stop immediately. He grabbed a Corelle mug from the cupboard, and then Papa, as we called him, drained the tuna juice into that mug. And then…he drank it. Drank. It. All. He said it was wasteful to throw out the liquid in which the tuna was packed.

With that gag-inducing memory relived in my head, the numerologist's words suddenly made sense. I was frugal by way of DNA. I had just forgotten or not really given it much thought. I loved spending money. But I could suddenly see his point.

He told me that, if I could ignore the pull to be frugal, the floodgates would open and riches would follow. He said the best way to ignore it was to live a little—to stop holding onto my money so tightly and splurge—because once I did, more money would pour in. *Um, dude, this session ain't cheap.*

Near the end of my short session, my numerologist asked what I did for a living. I had not previously mentioned it. I told him that I was a writer. He paused and looked at me and said, "Wow. I see nothing in your numbers that suggests you're remotely creative or a writer."

And then my time was up.

As I walked home, having hoped my numerology would inspire me, I was instead deflated and defeated, because I was, apparently, not a writer. Not anymore. Not according to the numbers. Problematic, since it was how I had been making my living and how I was going to pay for all this New Age stuff I'd just booked.

But I believed him. That night I tried to think of all the other things I could do instead. Nothing came to mind.

The very next day, waking up feeling desperate to figure out a new career and develop a new perspective on life, I decided I needed a break, so I went for Thai massage at seven in the morning. It was half-price at seven, so, okay, I was apparently even more frugal than I had thought but flexible about my schedule because I was a writer. But then I wasn't, so it was confusing.

In some back-alley-ish room, I let a stranger walk on my back, jam her elbows quite aggressively into my muscles, and pull on my arms in such a way that I felt like the wishbone on a cooked chicken. Strangely, when this Thai masseuse lady finished, she honked my breasts, like put one hand on each one and did a double squeeze—honk, honk. No other way to describe that, and I don't know why she did it. But it was weird.

Despite the bizarre and awkward ending, I felt relaxed afterward and was in a daze all morning. So I did what I never do and went home and napped, thereby proving what the numerologist had said: Morning Thai massages rendered me not a writer. Not that day, anyway. I was too tired to write. Thai massage became a weekly, er, twice-weekly thing over that six-week period. Okay, sometimes I went three times in a week, but it was steps from where I was living and half-price, so I was actually saving money.

I didn't get the boobie-honker again, though, which was an added bonus.

Everything's Coming Up Rainbows and Reiki

Next on my list: Reiki, a healing and relaxing Japanese ritual for moving energy around. I had considered trying Reiki before, but I'd been skeptical since the healer, as I understood it, never actually touched the patient. He or she just moved energy around, by magic, I guessed. That was initially difficult for me to wrap my head around.

But I had watched how it paid off in spades for Noah on *The Affair*. A little Reiki, and, one episode later, he went on to write an internationally revered blockbuster bestseller. It would surely work the same way for me, which would be double points because I'd have a bestseller *and* prove the numerologist wrong.

My friend Martha, who lived in Venice, knew of a practitioner who offered something similar to Reiki and who, according to Martha, had changed many people's lives with her services. I contacted said healer and learned that her technique was not traditional Reiki, but I was told the results would be similar.

Appointment booked, I was instructed via email to wear bright colors for my session. I had one pink T-shirt with red wine spilled down the front, so I wore that. With black Lululemon pants. That was as bright as I could muster, considering how strongly I apparently needed to protect myself with that black outfit shell.

The healer's studio was flush with rainbows. I therefore named her in my head the Rainbow Healer. The two-hundred-dollar-an-hour practitioner had each finger and toenail painted a different color of the rainbow, and rainbow paraphernalia hung on the walls as well. There were also feathery dreamcatchers (yeah, I know my spiritual accoutrement) and crystals hung all around the room. She could best be described as a modern hippie who, as the story goes, found her calling during an ayahuasca-fueled trip to Peru that had her seeing rainbows shoot from everywhere.

After an initial hello, she began shuffling the Tarot cards and then asked me what I wanted to work on. Before I opened myself up to her, I admitted that I was a major skeptic. With that off my chest, I told her that I was feeling stuck. If writer's block existed, I had it. I explained that I had spent most of my time of late reviewing the to-do list in my head and very little getting work done.

She said, "No problem."

As directed, I pulled a card from a deck. That card, Flowering, revealed that Zen wanted me living in abundance, in totality, living with intensity.

A theme was emerging.

Then, as directed, I hopped up on this woman's table, and she put her eyeballs almost right up to my eyeballs and stared so intensely that I felt panicked. I thought to myself, *If she honks my breasts, I'm leaving.* Then I lay down and breathed as I was told: two hard and deep breaths in, and one out, both through the mouth, which I did until I basically began to hyperventilate. Actually, even then, I continued.

As I remained still, save for the movement caused by my intense breathing, I listened to gongs and her peculiar chants, and my own air going in and out. Then suddenly, uncontrollably, after only fifteen minutes or so, I began to sob with such force I couldn't catch my breath. I sobbed. Big, ugly, soaking wet sobs, like the kind Viola Davis does when she wins an award. It was overwhelming to say the least, but mostly it was surprising.

That crying, I was told an hour later, was all the stuff inside me that needed to get out. Bad stuff and blocked energy in me was thick. She told me also that she'd had a strong mother vibe the entire time I was being treated.

"Yes, I was thinking about my mother," I said.

"Is she still with us?" she asked.

"She is. Is she going to die?" I asked.

"Yes, someday. We all are," she said.

I left feeling completely drained. Like more drained than I did the day I ran the New York Marathon. More drained than I had felt maybe ever. Lighter and clearer, sure, I felt that, too. But swollen-faced and drained. I slept for twelve hours that night and to be clear: I'm not a sleeper. If I can get in seven hours with just one middle-of-the-night wake-up, that's a win for me.

Rainbow-healing-energy-moving-take-on-Reiki: You had me at hello.

The healer had mentioned a recent client who had paid for the five-pack and knocked them all out in one week. Her intention was to meet the man of her dreams; by day three she had, and they were engaged within the month.

With such certain results, who was I to not walk to the Bank of America for a brick of cash? Obviously, I signed up for the five-pack.

By session two and then three, I learned I needed to say what I wanted to say, that, somehow, I was holding back on that. She could tell because my throat, my voice, was blocked. "I don't care," was no longer to be my standard answer when, for example, my friends asked what we should order at a restaurant. Or the times when I could do a favor that I really didn't want to or have time to do, but said yes anyway—I unknowingly (well, maybe knowingly) did that a lot. And the entire time, I had truly thought that I didn't care about little things.

But Rainbow Healing revealed that I actually did care. And that, when I let someone else make my decision for me, rather than voice my opinion, the result would always be a lot of time spent stewing in my head. I would stew and stew and stew. I was a stewer (I also make a very good beef stew, but I digress). And stewing caused clogging, and clogging needed releasing. Rainbow Healing was the emotional equivalent of having the drain snaked.

Later, I didn't quite execute on the "no" stuff, but I became more aware of it as a shortcoming. Having said that, I was inspired to write my mom a love letter. For no reason other than that I just felt like it after a session one day.

Also, I truly did suddenly feel clearer and more focused at the computer. I was not only getting work done but also writing some good stuff. I wondered, of course, by continuing with Rainbow Healing, was I simply paying someone to let me go sit in her house and cry? Maybe. But did it matter if it worked? All that junk needed to come out. If this healer could yank it from me, it was worth the cash.

By session four, the tables really began to turn. At one point during a session, as she was giving me my voice back with her movement of energy, it felt as though a twenty-pound flat weight was resting on my sternum. And then by the end of the session it was no longer there, though I didn't recall her lifting it off me. I asked her about that weight. She told me there was no weight, that was just pressure being lifted. I would have bet my house that something had been placed on my chest. I could have cheated and looked, but I didn't want to break the calm.

I wasn't drained when I left. Instead, this time, I was energized. I felt even more focused, and it was the first time I had an inkling of the notion that, if I could just remain calm and find peace in everything, I wouldn't feel so scattered. I felt equipped to set some boundaries with friends and even clients. Later that would falter, but I maintained an awareness of my habits in the months that followed, even as I struggled to keep them in place.

On that table, my mind would race a little. But, by the end of each of those last two sessions, I emerged with a mini-epiphany about one thing or another. And on session five, and I'm not making this up, for the first time in my life, I went into some sort of ultra-deep meditative zone. As I breathed, my breath became like a wave—rolling up to my head and then down to my toes. I was the ocean. I could physically feel it. Once I snapped out of that, my mind started racing and spinning like it usually does. But as my session came to a close, I kept thinking of myself splashing around in the ocean.

Something finally worked on my self-help quest. While I had previously thought of abandoning my efforts, it seemed like leaning in was a better option.

I'll Never Be Saved

A couple of weeks into that LA trip, I went to hear a friend speak at a party at someone else's house. Before I could enter, I was told by the host that first I had to be "saved." It reminded me of a conversation I'd had with a girl in high school with sparkly eyes, a bright smile, and curly hair, named Patty. She was a Bible lover. Not remotely as overt as those I'd meet later in life, who would Jesus-bomb me with group text Bible passages on the holidays, but she brought Jesus up in conversations the way I might have, at the time, brought up a trip to the mall.

She talked about Jesus and church in ways nobody else did at my public high school. One day, while we were eating lunch in the cafeteria, she told us that her family went to church more than just on Sundays. Over sandwiches that my frugal father had packed for me in recycled milk bags (in Canada, milk comes in bags), Patty explained to everyone at our table that Jesus Christ was our Savior (I didn't know what that meant, but I didn't dare ask).

She asked me what church my family went to.

"None," I explained. "I have never been baptized."

She was horrified, of course.

"If you've never been baptized, you will never be saved," she said.

I didn't know what that meant then (or now), but it was upsetting anyway. I was un-save-able. Nothing about that sounded positive.

It was so disturbing, it stuck with me even thirty-plus years later.

So, when this woman blocking entry to a party at a private home in LA told me I was finally, actually *about to be saved*, Patty immediately flashed into my mind. She had been wrong all along.

I was finally about to be saved in a stranger's driveway in West Hollywood. Praise the Lord!

Sadly, I had misheard. Unfortunately, I had to be *saged* before entering the house. Not saved. I didn't know what that meant either. But I quickly learned. The woman in charge had a bundle of dried, smoking, smoldering greens that she waved around my head and body. I learned it was dried sage. Sageing clears stuff out too, I was told.

I made a mental note to sage my house when I got back home. If I was to head back east all clear and revived, I didn't want to screw up all my efforts with an un-saged home.

A week later, on my way in to a Friday night Sound Bath Meditation, I found out I had to be *smudged* before going in. Like sageing, the woman standing at the entry to the yoga studio held a smoldering, red-embered bundle of dried stuff. I assumed that, by smudging, she meant she was going to wipe that thing on my forehead à la Ash Wednesday. I braced, hoping the burn wouldn't scar. But she started waving the smudge thing all over in the air. I knew what was happening. I knew sageing when I saw it.

"Am I being saged?" I asked, like a smug sage veteran.

"Yes," she said.

Sageing and smudging were one and the same. Who knew? I was getting saged all over LA, just like a local.

Once properly smudged-slash-saged, I paid forty-five dollars, then entered the studio on Rose Avenue for Sound Bath Meditation. I had dragged my friend Martha along with me (she had also done the five-pack Rainbow Healing). I assumed water would be involved, but I wasn't quite sure how, so I just wore yoga gear. As per the directions on the advertisement, I carried in a blanket, a yoga mat, and a little towel for my head. I thought I was well-prepared, but as I looked around at the rest of the floor upon entering the studio, I realized I looked like a total amateur.

Everyone had essentially moved their entire bedroom set into this studio. Pillows, bolsters, thick pads to lie on, the works. Martha and I set up our subpar napping equipment and settled in to be bathed.

As a group, we set our intentions, some people out loud, some of us in our heads, and then basically settled in for what ultimately felt like group Rainbow Healing. But with, apparently, pretty musical sounds from bowls.

Eyes closed, snuggled into my makeshift sleeping set-up, I couldn't have felt calmer. I'd just done an expedited five-pack of Rainbow Healing, so this was mostly a cherry on the top for me. Once things got underway and everybody began breathing, most of the rest of the room was suddenly an orchestra of tears and pained gasps.

Every once in a while, we were instructed to scream as loud as we could. That was startling and exhilarating all at once.

Eventually, the sound bath part started. There was a guy named Guy with loads of wavy light brown hair making beautiful sounds with all sorts of giant glass bowls and a gong. It was incredibly loud; you could feel the sound before you heard it. It was spellbinding and captivating.

The crying mostly stopped. Then a recording of a voice came on. I'm paraphrasing, but he said something like: If you have trouble knowing what you want, it's because you already have it. That resonated. I thought back to the recent billion-dollar lottery mania that had been happening at the time. I hadn't won, but I was okay with that.

I didn't hear much else this disembodied voice had to say because I eventually realized he sounded like L. Ron Hubbard of Scientology fame. It wasn't him, as far as I knew, but I got so obsessed with the voice that I was taken out of the peace and meditative nature of the sound bath. Also, I thought that— considering how seriously I was hitting the New Age stuff at this particular moment and how susceptible I was to believing it all—had the opportunity presented itself way back, I might very well have ended up in a cult, though my mother had often warned me before I left for college to stay away from the Moonies.

The sound bath lasted two hours. (And there was no water involved, so I was grateful I hadn't shown up in a bikini.) But the entire experience seemed like five minutes. I felt drugged at the end of it. Afterward I was in a strange and unrecognizable zone. I had found some peace (albeit fleeting), big-time.

Everyone described their experience out loud to the group. I couldn't move or open my mouth or open my eyes. I sat cross-legged for fifteen minutes, as still as I've ever sat in my lifetime. That stuff worked. Martha said she had the opposite reaction. She didn't feel calm, she felt terrified. She wanted to bolt from the room for the first half of things, and then she fell asleep and missed the sound bath completely.

Afterward, Martha said I might not be able to come to LA again because I was costing her too much money by making her join in on my Zen Bender. Though it was her idea for us to drive to Rama to get flowing white clothing for the next sound bath meditation. Wherever or whatever Rama was.

Celestial Cram

If you call the Spiritual Dove, she answers the phone, "Hello, it's the Spiritual Dove."

That alone was a strong selling point. That's deep commitment, sticking to what I'm certain was not her birth name. To add to that, when you meet her, she's an elegant woman with a British accent, and just listening to her talk is frankly quite calming.

I'd been told by a couple of people that the Spiritual Dove, a clairvoyant, knew everything. That her visions were incredibly detailed and that she didn't hold back. One person told me she learned of a cheating boyfriend via a session with the Spiritual Dove and was then given a vivid description of her future life that matched the one she'd dreamed of.

Bingo. I wanted to know what was coming. Who needed a vision board when the Spiritual Dove could get right down to it with her intuitive reading skills?

My first session with the Dove (that's what I call her for short) was amazing in its detail. She described the man I was going to meet in such specific terms it felt a certainty that we'd be together. The location (Orange County), where we were going to live (nice home, view of the ocean, but a few houses back from oceanfront), everything down to us holding cocktails as we chatted, watching a sunset.

The key identifying factor for this future husband of mine was that he was a widower. When I later described this session to my friend Layla, she said, "Widower, like we need to get a bus and take someone out with an 'accident,' or is the wife already gone?" Friends like Layla, willing to commit murder to find me a husband, are the kind we all need in our lives.

The latter, I learned, was the case. The wife was, according to the Dove, long gone, and this man was wandering around waiting for me because, according to the Dove, our life together was a done deal. It's been years and I have yet to find this guy, so I hope he's patient.

The other thing the Dove told me, which was not the first time I had been told this—and it turned out not to be the last—was that I would be world famous. That could have meant all sorts of things, of course—infamous, like I went crazy and went on a three-state crime spree, or perhaps got a little overzealous, like Layla implied, on the creating-a-widower situation, or I could do something great. Or write something great. Who knew?

Along with Mr. Widower, I'm still waiting for that fame and whatever was to follow.

So enthralled was I with the Dove that I, along with a bunch of friends, hired her later to come to my rented bungalow and tell me more. What she told me the second time wasn't so much different than what I had heard the first time.

That had to be good, right?

But, after my friend Martha emerged from her two-hundred-dollar session, she said, "You told her my life story ahead of time?"

Obviously, I had not.

The Dove knew so much about Martha, quite random details, it was jaw-dropping. Even if I had known the details about Martha that the Dove did, which I did not, I pointed out that I hadn't spent my two hundred dollars talking about, or even mentioning, Martha. But the Dove knew the kind of detail that makes you a believer.

And I think that's the crux of some of these things: take the thread you want to believe and, instead of living in a state of skepticism, live in a state of hope. Did I ever imagine I'd be world famous? Only the last time someone told me I would be. Did it make me feel optimistic about doing something significant in my life? Sure. Did I spend fewer hours watching *Scandal* to make that mark on the world? No.

Between Doves and Rainbows, I peppered my days with small, mind-clearing, soul-cleansing activities, in part because my list was snowballing with every person I spoke with. If I told one person about the sound bath effect, they countered with the sensory bath that changed their life; for every hyperventilation-inducing Rainbow Healing session, I was one-upped with a cryogenic pod story.

Which is how I learned I was supposed to find a labyrinth to walk. There were many in the city. Like, I literally Googled labyrinths in LA and was amazed by the choices. Supposedly, walking a labyrinth was a decision-making, head-clearing exercise, and coincidentally (or not) I needed to decide whether to pass or accept a project I had been mulling.

Undecided on which labyrinth to walk to decide on something else, fortunately, I stumbled across one near Electric Avenue in Venice while I was out for a regular walk. Serendipitous for certain. Without much thought, I entered the very basic maze mapped out in the grass with rocks. As I walked, I concentrated on the decision at hand. It was a quick walk, only a few minutes, but it gave me enough time to do some pros and cons.

The book in question was one I wanted to write. It sounded exciting, and it was for a celebrity I'd been a fan of. But the negotiations had gotten complicated and, for that matter, expensive too, as my lawyer was involved in the discussions. Never mind the labyrinth, my lawyer Liz had told me at the start to consider walking away from this potential deal. And she told me again in the middle. And she told me as it was all looking dire too, that maybe it wasn't going to work out. Still, I placed my decision-making in the labyrinth's hands, not my ass-kicking lawyer Liz who had always steered me right.

By the end of my quick walk, it appeared as though Liz and the labyrinth were on the same page. I decided to pass on the project, even though when I entered the labyrinth, I had *really* wanted to exit certain I should say yes to it. I also realized it would have been cheaper to have walked the labyrinth in the first place.

Not until much later did I notice a pattern had slowly been emerging. The more deeply I embraced the fixes offered up, the less I listened to my gut (and my lawyer). The labyrinth had helped me figure something out, but it was possibly something that I already knew.

Still, I was deep in by this point—any crutch, any guru. I wanted to relinquish my decision-making to those people and methods that surely had to be wiser than I.

Parched and decided, I continued on foot from the labyrinth to get juiced—Moon Juice, of course, on Rose Avenue, which is ground zero for serious juicers. Many people had told me to try it, so of course I did. I spent an hour choosing which twelve-dollar juice to buy. I went for an anxiety-reducing, calming one made with rose water and strawberries. But then I doubled down and got an energy-boosting, thyroid-bolstering one with carrot. I drank them both, back to back. I felt like Elvis, using uppers and downers all at once.

As a last-minute cram, before leaving LA that trip, I bought myself a set of Osho Zen Tarot cards, which I've pulled maybe five times in five years, and some dried sage. And while the card habit didn't stick, and I resumed my *I don't drink juice* policy (as per a nutritionist), I do sage my space with great regularity.

I even started calling my home "my space." How New Age was that?

Bottom line: I soaked up my healers' wisdom like a sponge. Only, looking back, I can admit it was too much all at once. But the energy work and the sound bath and the labyrinth, well, they were all meditation in one form or another. Thai massage, twice-a-week energy movement. And there was yoga that I went to on a regular schedule too, and that helped. Here's the other thing: I had created, in that short period of time, a routine. Routine can lull a crazy mind. Empty, unscheduled space in a day can make the head stir in wild ways.

Maybe suddenly working from home, after so many years in an often raucous, social, and buzzy newsroom, played a role in my off-the-rails spiritual pursuit as well, because it took me a while to figure out how to manage the endless sea of unbooked time that only I could schedule.

To fill the new slate of time I had open in front of me, I tackled a lot of non-work projects and replaced the social aspect of life that I was missing from working in a newsroom with…well, anything I could find. In Venice Beach, I liked the appointments. They gave me a schedule to stick to.

Did it all reduce my anxiety? Well, yes, absolutely, for a short time while I was there, but it also caused some. I spent close to $1,800 on all my advisors and elixirs.

That part actually stressed me out and made me wonder if, in fact, I did have more money than brains. But despite the drain on my bank account, I felt clearer, sharper, lighter, and maybe more laid-back. I'm not super easy-going, as most people who know me can attest, so that was a plus.

Did the sun shining brightly on that coast help? Most certainly. Was the slow pace and hippie vibe of Venice contagious? Absolutely.

My Rainbow Healer told me, in the future, when I got distracted or anxious or whatever, to remember my intention: finding peace. I felt peaceful. Would it last? I pondered that as I put on my black jeans, black boots, black sweater, and black leather jacket and headed out to catch a plane, back to the chaos I loved.

Amid that black shell, I tucked a red piece of crystal one healer had given me into my pocket as I traveled. It was a security blanket—a tiny takeaway from a rapid-fire, accelerated journey to an enlightened state. Would it work? To find our own internal strength and power and clear out the cobwebs, maybe we just have to believe it is possible. I learned that you have to weed out the crazy stuff, and listen to what's positive and resonates for you. A healthy dose of spirituality, reflection, and looking inward stills my mind. That I can take with me anywhere, for free, any time.

Plus, my Rainbow Healer assured me that, if I slipped up, she could always do energy work over Skype.

CHAPTER 6

THE MELROSE PLACE OF IT ALL

anxiety

When I first moved to Harlem, I was walking uptown to see a friend who lived about twenty blocks north of me. It was a clear and sunny but brisk winter day, so I was moving quickly up a bustling avenue. A guy passing by said, "What up, Snowflake?"

I slowed to look back at him, but he was continuing and didn't look back at all. I mulled his words as I continued my trip, not sure I'd heard him correctly, and not sure what he'd said was actually directed toward me. But then, not a block later, another guy said the exact same thing—"What up, Snowflake?"—and this time, clearly it was said to me. I was stopped at the light, waiting to walk across, and so was he. Eye contact was made.

I was Snowflake.

Why was everybody calling me Snowflake? I truly had no idea.

Could it have been because everyone somehow knew I was from Canada? That was my initial thought. It had to have been that. But how could anyone know I was Canadian? I quickly scanned my outfit, felt my hat to see which one I was wearing, and checked the bag I was carrying to see if anywhere on me was a flag or a maple leaf or some indication that I liked Tim Hortons. Nothing. I was perplexed.

Eventually, as I continued on my way, I decided that I was being called "snowflake" because I was wearing a super bright pink puffy coat with a faux-fur collar. It had to be that. These guys were making fun of my bright outerwear. It made perfect sense. It wasn't snowing at the time, so maybe the implication was that I was overdressed and waiting for snowflakes. That made the most sense.

When I got home, still pondering my experience, I Googled "snowflake" to learn that it wasn't at all about my puffy pink jacket, but rather my pale white skin.

Fascinated and fully entertained, I had a good chuckle at both my complete lack of knowledge and my total un-cool-ness, as well as at how amusing the experience had been. But it also reinforced for me something that had originally caused me some grief when I first closed on my apartment. I was an evil *gentrifier*, and that didn't feel good.

Fire Escape in My Igloo

While my Harlem time was filled with many only-in-Harlem happenings, and some exceptional and lifelong friendships were formed, a lot of soul-searching and Zen Bendering went down while I lived there. Mostly because, for me, living there represented the Great Recession. That's where I was when I lost my job. In fact, I vividly remember, just before the layoff, mentioning at a building board meeting that I had been reading about people getting laid off and not being able to pay their condo and co-op fees, and that buildings, as a result, were going bankrupt. I said that someone in our building could indeed find themselves unemployed, so we should keep our reserves flush.

It didn't strike me that I'd be first to find myself in that situation.

I was the first and, for a while, only, until eventually there were four of us in the building who had lost our jobs. Strangely, that turned out to be a positive in a messy situation. Later, when I collaborated on *The Loving Diet*, by Jessica Flanigan, the main premise of her book (though it referred to illness) was that we should love our way through adversity and find an upside to help us heal. The four of us at Casa Loma (the strange name for our building, which we edited in conversations to Casa Loco) who were home all day began to do potluck, rooftop lunches. I was too deep in it to see it at the time, but those group lunches were uplifting. They were the upside. They were an amazing break from rocking back and forth in a ball in tears on the floor of my apartment, and it was nice to have some similarly troubled people to commiserate with.

When I lived there, a lot of new construction was happening all around, much of which had begun in the optimistic boom years of 2006 and 2007, and some of it was halted completely or slowed. Along with everybody in my building on West 116th Street, I had bought in 2007—right at the height of the market. That was in part because a fancy condo building on Central Park North had just fetched the highest price per square foot above

96th Street (even though it was a few doors down from a prison, albeit a prison with a view of the park), and that set the tone for neighborhood pricing to follow.

Pricing to follow before the real estate market nearly plunged into the abyss one year later. Translation: Everyone in my building paid the maximum possible dollar per square foot to live in our little five-story, sixteen-apartment complex—we all bought right at the apex—so, that was super good fortune. And then for a long time, despite job loss and career change, selling wasn't an option without a loss. And I wasn't taking a loss.

I had bought and sold real estate before, just not in New York City. But in some sort of momentary lapse in judgment, I made a hasty purchase. Owning in New York comes with a long list of challenges unique to the city, and to shared living in general.

Plus, I hadn't really looked around too much to investigate various neighborhoods. I had checked out an apartment here or there, three tops, altogether. So, while I was renting in a rather convenient neighborhood at 59th and Columbus and loving it, I somehow felt I was built and fully equipped for owning an apartment in New York and all the stress that came along with it.

As such, I viewed the apartment once for about fifteen minutes, then, when I got home, I put in a bid to buy it. And that bid was accepted. And that was it.

To put this in perspective, I spent six days researching what type of television to buy. And six to twelve minutes debating a Manhattan real-estate transaction.

There were multiple challenges I hadn't considered, including distance from a lot of my usual New York action. When I had to go to a midtown office, it was a thirty-minute subway ride (compared to my previous ten-minute walk), but if I was going to the gym and then out for the evening, I felt compelled to lug bags of costume changes around the city with me, rather than waste thirty minutes going uptown to change and thirty minutes or more to head back down. And when I came home late at night, I quickly learned that a taxi to 116th Street cost substantially more than one to 59th street. Uptown felt very far and out of the way and therefore very inconvenient.

Additionally, I loved to walk at night in New York. It's still one of my favorite things to do. But not knowing the area well, and perhaps being nervous about the emptiness and the quietness of the streets, plus what I had read about the crime rate (which in fairness was not much different from most neighborhoods in New York), I stopped doing my all-time favorite activity.

To add to that, while there was an initial dorm-room feel to living in that building, and we all got to know one another as neighbors by socializing on the roof and visiting one another's apartments with regularity (a very un-New-York-like practice), eventually there was a lot of infighting. That's because owning in New York meant co-owning public space. Co-owning space meant co-making decisions about that space. We all owned a piece of the hallways, and the stairs, and the rooftop, which, as it turned out at Casa Loco, meant that when a group decision needed to be made, war often ensued.

So you understand how ugly it got at times: Once, a neighbor referred to me as a "cow" on Facebook for asking them to be quiet, to which someone on the chain commented that my neighbor should "teach that cow a lesson." This didn't feel like normal warfare.

In one battle royal over putting a couch on the roof (which was preceded by wars over dogs on the roof, flowers on the roof, and party hours on the roof), things got particularly ugly. Teams formed. Factions emerged. There was a clear divide between sides. There were no fence-sitters in this particular war and no middle ground. Couch. No couch. Period.

There was the rational group (no couch) and the irrational one (pro-couch). During Couchgate, names were suddenly being called, and vicious emails were fired off.

There were many ugly situations, but a crescendo of sorts was reached when someone left a Spanx catalogue at the door of the female board president. Though a breaking point had been coming for a long time, that war and the tactics used to fight it led to utter dead-to-me silence in the hallways or on the roof. Icing the other team, fully and unapologetically, became standard operating procedure. I could very easily walk right by someone from the other side and make no eye contact and not say a word. Zero discomfort. Zero regret. And so could they. Elevator rides weren't just chilly, they were downright frigid.

It wasn't just the fighting that made home not fun; I was stressed-out from the second I moved into Casa Loco, and then, a year later, mega-twisted when I lost my job, which made the infighting, my job circumstance, and the neighborhood merge into one so that, most of the time, almost from the beginning, all I could think of was leaving. The apartment itself became guilty by association. I was one foot out the door, constantly planning an escape or maybe always looking for something better.

When I was a kid, my dad used to shovel snow into a giant pile and then dig the inside out so we had a snow fort. Wrapped in bright stiff snowsuits, suffocating from tightly tied thick, wide, and colorful scarves my grandmother had knit, we played outside in those forts for hours. It was like having a tree fort, but on the ground in igloo form.

Each time my dad made us a fort, he would do the strangest thing. He would carve out both a front door and a back door, then he would explain that the back door was a fire escape.

Keep in mind, none of us played with matches. But then who didn't remember that *Little House on the Prairie* episode in which Mary dropped her glasses in the field after her horse-drawn cart got toppled and the magnification of the lenses lit the grass up in flames? I never did ask about the odds of flames erupting in the cold igloo.

Once, when my neighbor, also named Stefanie (but with an "f"), and I were young, we were making fun of another kid on the street and his girlfriend. (I'm embarrassed to say, we called her ugly.) That's what we did back then, I guess (along with singing Anne Murray songs in the rec room). He got so mad he started chasing us down the street. We were in snowsuits and the street was deep in snow and ice, so we ran as fast as we could to get away, but it wasn't easy to escape. We made it to her backyard and dove into her snow fort. He caught up to us and eventually made his way to the igloo door. He hunched down and started yelling at us for being mean. I was terrified.

And there was no fire escape in her igloo. We were trapped.

That's how I felt in Harlem, thanks to the real estate market and my fellow apartment owners. Trapped.

Home Was Never My Sanctuary

Years before moving to Harlem, I injured my arm and shoulder. Physical therapy helped, but acupuncture was the big fix in the end. A referral from a friend led me to a practitioner named Alexis Arvidson. Later, when I couldn't sleep and was a total stress bag, I read about the calming effects of the ancient Chinese remedy that involved microneedles and pressure points and something called chi, and so I decided to return to Alexis, who had saved my bicep, to see if she could also save my sanity.

Alexis, like all good healers, had a studio with a feathered dreamcatcher and crystals and oils all around. Calming spa-type music and mood lighting eased my tension upon entering, but not as much as Alexis' presence did. She's got a special vibe all her own. As directed, I hopped up on her table and let her do her magic. Despite a paralyzing fear of needles in general, I found acupuncture soothing. And, after learning that chi was energy, and that Alexis was moving mine around, I also discovered that the ritual helped me sleep and chilled me out, even if only for a fleeting moment.

After one visit, I was sold.

I began to go monthly when I could. And Alexis became the de facto head of my wellness team. I began to treat acupuncture as my preventive medicine splurge, plus she cured my iPhone-itis (as in my wrist and elbow throbbed from texting and social media-ing). She helped with my lower back issues, headaches, whatever. During my monthly visits, she was (and continues to be) on it.

Interestingly, Alexis didn't just deal with my chi. She pulled out anatomy books, discussed injuries, talked about emotional issues, and we chitchatted too—discussing personal finance, politics, the perils of homeownership, ticks, life in the era of Trump, and of course self-help books. She practiced alternative medicine, but she offered up a well-rounded approach to physical and mental health. Like me and most people I know, she's only about 10 percent out there, if you know what I mean by that. Not outer space out there. Just New Age out there. And I like that out-there side of her. But I also like that she's grounded in reality and has never steered me wrong.

She and I would discuss whatever crisis du jour was going on in my life, as I lay on her table with needles sticking out of my legs, feet, ears, and stomach, and we would talk through my stress. One day, she made a rather astute observation: that most situations that caused me anxiety could in some way be traced back to my home. That home was not a sanctuary for me. In fact, it had become a torture chamber.

The more I thought about it, the more I realized that she was right. Even sharing with her some events that pre-dated Harlem, home had been a cause for anxiety, for one reason or another.

When she first brought it up, I didn't have an answer, and she didn't have an immediate solution, but it did start me thinking.

At the time, I was also collaborating on a book called *You Are WHY You Eat*, by Dr. Ramani Durvasula. Dr. Ramani always gave me so much good advice, and I gleaned a lot of it editing her writing. As we talked through a lot of the notions in her book, the idea of the stakes getting higher in certain situations started to resonate with me. I was working for myself. I was becoming aware of age, and life, and the fact that time wasn't infinite. And so, the stakes were higher. I wasn't twenty. Parents were aging, retirement was looming, and things I'd once not given a care about were front and center on my worry list.

Dr. Ramani's book wasn't about eating alone, or really about eating at all, though it shed interesting light on the concept of eating to please other people and struggles with weight. More, it addressed the concept of tackling weight problems in order to empower yourself to tackle greater change in your life. Especially as the stakes soared.

All of it applied to my home situation. Dr. Ramani's theory on my home choice was an interesting one: She felt that, by choosing the actual structure in which I lived as a priority over the neighborhood that it stood in, I had made certain assumptions about myself that were completely incorrect. And in doing so, I had forced something on myself that I didn't like, and therefore put myself in a bad mood that never went away.

She was correct in many ways.

I had made my purchase in the dead of winter, when the streets were quiet. At the time, I didn't notice or predict that this would be an important factor. But when the spring and summer months rolled around and the sun was shining, when the wonders of the streets of New York came alive, a cacophony of humanity took to 116th and it came alive with gatherings and social interaction that I hadn't expected, that in the evening proved lovely, but in the day proved distracting for a stay-at-home writer.

Additionally, at the time of purchase, I was leaving for work each day, and, while things like local wine stores and yoga studios didn't seem important because I knew those conveniences were a mere subway ride away, later, when I was working from home, it would have come in handy if they had been within walking distance. (They both eventually popped up in the neighborhood but, patience not being my strong suit, I had by then become frazzled over the lack of either.)

Most of my assumptions about my needs and what I wanted proved very wrong and, indeed, extremely problematic. I needed quiet. I needed convenience, like being close enough to the action that I craved.

Apparently, I didn't know myself very well. I didn't know what would bother me. But Dr. Ramani did.

What I didn't know was that I didn't need a big space. That meant I had made an erroneous compromise. New York City is full of trade-offs. But when it came to living, I had made one that was too big for me to handle. I thought I wanted a larger apartment, so I made a classic New York choice—location versus size. I chose wrong.

After seven years in Harlem, and the insights of Alexis and Dr. Ramani, I finally realized that size didn't actually matter.

Like shiny hair, neither did shiny marble countertops or Kohler faucets. What mattered to me was peace, which wasn't happening inside my building, and it wasn't happening on my street when I stepped out.

It took me some time to figure out how to change my situation. Though seemingly unrelated, I began by doing what Dr. Ramani said to do on many fronts. I started eating on small plates. I started watching the way people would encourage me to eat or drink with them (to feel better about their own eating habits, they needed someone to eat or drink as much as they did), and maybe most importantly, I started to at least notice when I didn't trust my gut, or, as she called it, "spider senses." I started taking note of the stakes and which ones rose and which ones mattered most.

All these small moves started to bring an awareness to my life that I hadn't possessed before. I realized that I spun on a daily basis. And I chased my life, rather than living it in a more conscious way.

Dr. Ramani theorized that our initial feeling on something is often spot-on, but that, at times, we get ourselves deeper into situations even though they feel wrong; as we do, the stakes get higher, and extricating ourselves becomes more difficult. Taking all those smaller steps, as Dr. Ramani suggested, empowered me to see clearly about a larger one.

That was my home life. Eventually, I could see that situation very clearly. Not only was it too expensive for the income I was then suddenly not bringing in, but also it was too stressful—and too full of compromise.

Seven years after moving in, my neighbor Doug got a job in Los Angeles and put his Harlem apartment one floor below mine on the market. Within twenty-four hours, he had seven offers.

The recession was over. And so was my time in Harlem.

I listed my apartment, and without having anywhere to go, I jumped once again, hoping a net would form. I put my things in storage and checked out of Casa Loco. Like my decision to quit my job, I had a solid positive vibe about my move, though I had no real plan.

Something else happened once I knew I was leaving. I started feeling okay about walking at night again. Late at night, I strolled the streets, keeping to the busier ones, feeling calmer and almost sorry to be leaving. It hadn't been the streets that were the problem, it had been my general high level of stress about my life situation that had kept me from stepping outside and doing what de-stressed me the most.

I realized during those walks: I didn't want to leave New York. I wanted to leave a building that had grown too chaotic for my state of mind. It was a fun place to live once, but then it wasn't. Leaving was a risk. I might never make it back to the city I loved. But then again, I'd been pretty clear on that vision board that the city was part of my way of life.

Dramatically less expensive, with small, manageable compromises, three months after moving out, I closed on a simple house in Springs in the Hamptons. A valuable lesson was learned: Life will always be full of compromise. The key is to know ourselves enough to figure out which ones we can best manage.

Looking at this in the rearview mirror, I eventually saw another by-product of following Dr. Ramani's book. Fear, in many ways, was slowly starting to leave me.

Many people have at times told me I am brave. I would have described myself more as bold, as I think I'm chicken about a lot of things. After constant warnings as a child against talking to strangers, I'll admit I'm still worried about getting kidnapped, like everyone was all the time in the after-school specials. There still exists that genuine fear of getting my head taken off by a Sears truck, like my mother always warned.

But once again, I took a chance and made a step to finding some peace. For every five failed fixes I had tried, a couple of them had finally worked.

◐

CHAPTER 7

THE LIFE-CHANGING MAGIC OF TAPPING INTO AN OBSESSIVE-COMPULSIVE DISORDER YOU DIDN'T KNOW YOU HAD

home

If you've ever struggled with weight, you know the shame and frustration of never finding anything to wear. It's really occupied so much of my headspace that, if never being able to find clothes that fit was my job, I'd be rich and would have been able to retire long ago.

What could I have accomplished if I had used the time more wisely, instead of always stressing about what was in my closet that would look the least bad? Probably a lot.

I was nominated for a New York Emmy for a reality show I had created, but I didn't go to the ceremony because I was so worried about finding something to wear. I knew I'd be uncomfortable, as I was challenging to fit, so instead I didn't even try—I decided to avoid the agony of shopping and pretend I was above going, that it wasn't important to me. Oddly enough, I had just won a raffle, something I was prone to doing, for a custom-made gown. Even that didn't give me enough of a boost to go.

It's quite fair to say, that battle, both in my head and in my closet, has been the domineering force and utter brutal time-suck of my life. Period.

Part of the problem is that I'm short. If you're five foot two, I guarantee you've spent a considerable amount of your income having pants and sleeves and skirts shortened to accommodate your lack of height. In the olden days, there was no such thing as buying a pair of jeans and immediately wearing them. That changed at some point, as retailers started to sell tall, regular, and short jeans. Back in the day, a week's notice was required before wearing; jeans had to be purchased, washed, and shortened. Skirts, too. Dresses. Jackets. Everything.

Eventually, retailers and designers got savvy and offered a petite line for shorties like me. It was slow going at first—only a few places sold them. Though nobody ever offered a full line-up of height-challenged clothing, some retailers made some pieces available in a pinch. I always theorized that, as with sizes 10, 12, and 14, designers didn't want to see short or chubby people in their beautiful threads.

Ever walk into a store and have the clerk say, "We have more sizes in the back?" That means more sizes for the sturdier people. They only rack the tiny stuff so as to humiliate you into knowing you aren't front-of-store-worthy. I was told by a friend that the small ones come out of the box first, hence the back room for larger sizes, but still, if a scrawny clerk says that before I have even asked a question, she's sized me up.

I can't be certain, but in my '90s and 2000s world, Ann Taylor was one of the first to offer short-people clothing. Not that they were overly fashion forward (not that I was or am either), but there were basics, as a fashionista might say—cardigans, black and gray pants, shirts—the stuff people could wear every day with a little mixing and matching of accessories. That meant, as petite items went, it was Ann Taylor or the tailor.

Rarely did I need a suit for my job—in television, the well-dressed people were on air, and then there were the rest of us. The divide was clear and apparent. These days, working from home, if I get out of my pajamas by five in the afternoon, it's a fancy day at the office. I have regular Lululemon and dressier Lululemon for when I need to leave the compound and go to, say, the post office. If I had some sort of meeting back in the job days, then I would buy what I needed as I needed it. I was never a clothes horse.

On some occasion or other, I needed a summery suit. I don't recall why. I'm sure I had a black blazer and black pants, but for whatever reason, I needed a lighter option. A little thicker in the middle, bustier, I didn't always fit into the petite line exactly. It wasn't until years later, as boob jobs became mainstream, that designers started letting out the tops, which eventually gave me at least a fighting chance at buttoning a blazer.

Off to Ann Taylor on this specific occasion, I tried on eighty-two things and had my standard breakdown in the changing room, as I always did when I tried to find something to wear, before settling on a suit out of my price range (which was often what ended my meltdown—the clear decision to spend more than I should on fewer pieces to get out of there slightly less scathed and have one thing to wear).

That suit was gray with a single row of buttons. No shoulder pads. It had pinstripes in a gold-but-not-metallic color and white. The suit wasn't shiny, but it wasn't dull. The pants were the right length and proportion, but they zipped up at the side. None of this style was my best look; however, the jacket covered up the flaws. I was stuck with a compromise, as usual, but it was good enough.

I wore the suit once, for whatever I needed to wear it for. And then I hung it back in the closet with the rest of the one-timers that collected shoulder dust, glad to be out of it and hopeful I'd never have to see it again. Looking at it as it hung felt like failure; failure to be the right size and to find the right suit.

Years later, I needed a summer suit again. I had a job interview. At the time, my mother was visiting at my apartment at 59th and Columbus. Previously I had been able to suffer the indignity of tearing every single last item of clothing out of my closet in a desperate search to find one thing, anything, that fit or looked semi-okay, alone. I didn't have to share the horror episodes with anyone.

I tore through everything to find an interview suit. Closet almost empty, contents on the bed and floor, I found the Ann Taylor pinstripe option and zipped it up. I stepped out of my bedroom to check the full-length mirror in the hall, and my mother pointed out what I already knew, but was hoping wasn't apparent: The suit was tight.

That was being kind. The suit didn't fit.

My mother said very gently, "I think it's pulling a bit in the back."

So, when my poor unassuming mother, who would do anything on the planet to make me feel better and have an easy life, said something that was 100 percent true and that I already knew, I snapped at her. Looking back, "snapped" feels like an understatement.

"Unleashed" more aptly describes it.

I tore her head off. I felt, for one brief second, nothing but rage toward her, as though decades of anger about my ups and downs on the scale suddenly bubbled up and were her fault. As if having cried in my closet all those times I struggled hadn't let out the frustration, the remnants of every closet or retail-dressing-room fight leaked out of my pores at that very moment.

Logically, I knew it wasn't her fault that my ugly suit didn't fit. But I didn't want to hear it. *It* was already screaming inside my head in the same way it had every other time something didn't fit.

These are your damn genes. That's what I thought, not said.

Instead, I screamed at her in a rather unkind way some other words about not telling me what to do. Basically, in that horrible way one can only scream at one's mother, saying nothing that makes any sense, just using a ton of words to misdirect one's anger toward the one person who will tolerate it.

Uncharacteristically, I flipped out, which was not my typical behavior toward my mother.

And then, ten minutes later, my mother still liked me, for some strange reason.

I don't remember if I went out and bought a new suit for that interview, after blaming my mother for everything in my life, or if I squeezed in and squeezed by, but I clearly remember how ashamed I felt for not being able to zip that suit up, yes, but more for how I had misdirected my rage. I felt bad about it immediately and have ever since. I suspect that my mother, having raised three girls with short fuses, didn't even rank it in the top five irrational-child episodes of her life as a mom. Maybe she doesn't remember it. But I do.

Like every piece of shitty clothing in my wardrobe, that stupid suit survived various homes that I have lived in. I moved it with me from place to place. And I moved a lot. Each time, I dragged all my crap with me.

Along the way, my purges were always minimal. I had a system. I'd take a few items out of the closet that I hadn't worn in a couple of years and put them in a bag for Goodwill. Then I'd grab half of them back out of the bag, because it felt wasteful to toss a perfectly good dress circa 1994 that I'd never, ever, ever wear again, and so I'd pay money to have it moved along with my stuff. Every time.

Permission to Purge

Adulthood is often marked by the day one eliminates the last piece of college Ikea furniture from one's décor, though Ikea is making a decorating comeback as frugal becomes the new flashy, but for whatever reason, clothing didn't go the way of the standard-issue POÄNG chair everyone I knew in my twenties (including me) owned.

There were some clothing items I was nostalgic about, so I kept. I had a white blouse that always reminded me of a fun New York night—the time a random selection of work friends and I went for a drink, then spontaneously went to a club, then went to the Empire Diner and sat next to Sean Penn and ate blue-cheese burgers at five in the morning (and the entire night I stressed out because I'd left my first-floor bedroom window in Hoboken cracked ever so slightly, and FYI that apartment was eventually robbed).

My checkered crop pants reminded me of a fun trip I had with my younger sister, so I kept them even though they never even remotely fit after that trip. I have held onto a dress I wore once after hitting Weight Watchers so hard that I dropped so much weight it was unmaintainable. I kept that dress to stare at as aspiration for the next diet. Sometimes I kept things because, yes, they fit once. But due to my frugality or nostalgia or hope, I often hung on for too long.

Researching ideas for a book I had to write for someone who had compared her methodology to that of Marie Kondo, I read the blockbuster hit *The Life-Changing Magic of Tidying Up: The Japanese Art of Decluttering and Organizing.*

It didn't just help me clarify the work project at hand. I had settled into my home and was feeling more at peace there than anywhere I'd previously lived. That inspired me to make it even better by decluttering the space and therefore my life. And I was fully drawn in by the life-altering promise that good stuff would follow.

Plus, I had a permission slip to throw away as much as I wanted.

If you haven't read the book, the premise is really quite simple. If something doesn't spark joy, toss it. Period. If it brings you joy, keep it.

Marie Kondo's theory runs counter to many organizing books that don't take joy into account, but rather suggest, if you don't use it, toss it.

I do nothing half-assed. I read Marie Kondo's book, then took basically two full weeks or more off work (thereby pushing retirement further out of reach). But I had to. I had to follow her direction to the letter. After all, greatness was waiting.

As directed, I started with the small-ticket items, meaning the least emotionally charged ones, like clothing. I took every single item of clothing out of my closet, including outerwear and footwear, and I piled it high on the floor in one room. Then I held a piece up and decided whether it brought me joy. If it did, I kept it. Even if I had not worn it for years. If it did not, I garbaged it, donated it, sold it, but not before I closed my eyes and thanked it for its service. That's what Marie told me to do.

Once the burden of letting go of that one pair of jeans that I had shortened before washing (which turned them into floods) was lifted, doors would surely open. Hanging on to the torn pink T-shirt from J. Crew that I was wearing in Harlem when some guy said, "What up, Juicy Fruit?" was okay. It brought me continued joy because it made me laugh to think about. Surely leaving it rolled, not folded and stacked, in my drawer would force my dreams to come true.

And tossing that gray suit, that actually made me feel so incredibly gutted for yelling at my mom, felt downright liberating. I felt fireworks-exploding-in-my-bedroom kind of joy.

Keeping it pissed me off.

The question after it was all over: Why had I needed Marie Kondo's permission to get rid of any of it? Same reason we use all the self-help books—I wasn't alone. Hundreds of thousands of other people probably wanted to throw stuff out too, but felt bad about it.

And, of course, that promise—that life-altering promise that there's more out there. And it will be better than it was before you came home every day and emptied your handbag, then thanked it for a hard day.

Most of the rest of the KonMari system got done over the weeks that followed the clothing purge. I whittled my books down, not to thirty as directed, but I got rid of a lot. (*How to Put on a Fine Afternoon Tea* seemed not a keeper.) There wasn't much excess in my kitchen, but what did get pulled just got moved to clutter my basement.

Marie Kondo suggested a full clearing of all cosmetic samples. Initially, as a rule-follower, I did as I was told (not with Crème de la Mer samples, however; that's downright against the law and if it's not, it should be) and did a full sweep of all the travel-size shampoos and such. Looking back at my decluttering initiative, I understood her point.

Then I met Birchbox, one of the great true loves of my life. That company sends you samples every month. Before I knew it, my bathroom was joyfully recluttered with tiny squeeze bottles and mini mascaras. If Marie Kondo ever looked below my sink, she would sob. I stand behind that decision and realize that is the single shortcoming of the book that has changed sock drawers worldwide forever.

Birchbox 1 Kondo 0

But, as I dug into the stacks of photos and it became clear that I didn't need eleven photos of a snowy mountain that I couldn't identify, nor did I need photos of people skiing whose names I didn't even know, I made it a point to keep a picture or two of something that at one time was amusing. Admittedly, I got slowed down on this stuff (like she said I would), taking time to photograph the old photos and upload them to Facebook and create digital clutter in my phone.

Deep in the piles, I found a stack of photos from a Halloween party I had held in Hoboken in what had to be the mid-nineties. It sparked great joy.

In the photos, I was dressed as Carmen Miranda, and the photo made clear that my costume construction looked good, but I certainly had not taken engineering into account. I recalled as I looked at the photo that that tall tower of fruit on my head was painfully heavy and I likely slipped a disk or something wearing it. The photos also reminded me of an incident from that night. Someone had invited a cousin. And that cousin brought six friends. And those friends, as I recall, were state troopers. One of them picked up lasagna with his hands, which prompted the maker of the lasagna to say, "Lasagna isn't finger food." It's a bit of a blur, but, thanks to Lasagnagate, the troopers were asked to leave the party, which they did, for thirty-six seconds until the door of my tiny first-floor apartment burst back open, tables and papers at the door flying everywhere. A scuffle ensued, and it took a few people to eject the group of six—constricting costumes flying off in an effort to contain the situation. It was chaotic and stressful, but the lasagna lived and so did we.

Likely drunk, we all went on with the evening like it never happened. Those photos were keepers.

The greatest joy of Kondoing, once I had tossed most of everything I owned, was her permission slip to reorganize my remaining items as I saw fit. I liked that notion. I made myself an official sunglasses drawer at my front door because that worked for me. My clever niece, Kate, found it quite amusing when I referred to it as such. Sunglasses always fit, even when I gained five pounds. So it was a crowded drawer. Next to it I loaded a drawer with paint samples, fabric samples, and rug samples. This would probably be a weird configuration for others, but it worked for me.

And Kondo said that was okay.

The Dark Side to Marie Kondoing Your Home

To be clear, I went so far as to Kondo my freezer. And that shouldn't be written in the past tense, because I continue to keep it that way.

Consumed by Marie Kondo best describes what happened to me after reading her book. I was able to avoid working, and basically all else, for weeks while I knocked it out which, in hindsight, was a little obsessive. I had a can't-stop-won't-stop mentality, which was shockingly overwhelming.

I Kondoed hard.

And, honestly, I don't know how anyone could properly Kondo if they had to go to an office every single day.

The bigger problem, of course, was that I was left with almost nothing. I got carried away. Apparently, most everything I owned did not bring me joy. In fact, I was able to clear out fully four closets in my house. I have one in my bedroom so sparsely populated there is more empty shelf space than clothing, with about half a foot between each hanger.

Which of course made me wonder why I had settled on surrounding myself with things I didn't like. I'm not sure exactly. Perhaps my clothes were like vegetables, not dessert. I bought them because I needed them, but never really liked them.

Dr. Ramani's theory, when I asked her why I might have bought so much stuff I hated, was that numbing is numbing. Like food, shopping is a distraction that feeds us in the same way.

Whatever the underlying reason, much of it caused me so much struggle to zip up, I usually ended up hating it immediately.

The obvious question: Was it the clothing that I hated, or was it what I saw in the mirror?

Strangely, the Marc by Marc Jacobs five-hundred-dollar layoff bag lived to see another day. I didn't purge that. That bag sparked joy then and to this day. And it always fit.

Having said that, a desire to wear that stupid suit, or most everything else I owned, never did reemerge. There's an occasional scramble to find the odd belt, and I concede that I still have some little piles of costume jewelry or accessories to Kondo, but I don't regret tossing anything.

Sadly, I might have accidentally thrown a document in the garbage that I had saved for years. It was a letter from 1997, praising my work on a project. It had been written by a legendary journalist, and it indeed brought me great joy. A couple of years after the initial Kondo, I was having a conversation with a colleague who reminded me of it, so I went on a search to find it.

Search is the wrong word. I tore my entire house apart looking for it—to no avail. I hadn't thrown away the certificate that says I passed driver's education when I was sixteen. I had a full stack of emails and notes, including rejections, but not the coveted one I wanted to find. I would never have thrown it away, but, in my Kondo fury, well, it must have gotten shredded or fireplaced. Or else, someday, somewhere, I'll find it, just like I did the title to my house after a one-week search, and the slip of paper that provided evidence that I had served jury duty for fourteen days.

Or it's gone. And if it's gone, I will blame Ms. Kondo. There were so many stacks and stacks of stuff, it's not a stretch to think that a rogue slice of paper might have slipped into the wrong pile.

Another problem that emerged: Once I Kondoed, when things got un-Kondoed, I came a little unglued.

And when that happened, I found myself unable to get much done until I re-Kondoed a drawer or pile. The un-Kondoed items sparked angst, creating a vicious cycle of work and sock-rolling and handbag-stuffing, ping-ponging me between joy and stress almost weekly.

In fact, my obsession with keeping everything Kondoed grew constant and overwhelming. When my sock drawer got messed up, I got a little spun.

It's one thing to Kondo, it's another to *maintain a full Kondo order.*

Shonda Rhymes explained, in her book *The Year of Yes*, that she can't sit down to write until everything else is done. I can relate. It's so much easier to whip through the to-do list than to write. And that to-do list grows most days, rather than shrinks. Marie

Kondo's way of life became an ongoing never-ending to-do on the list, adding an extra layer of work to a day already rife with procrastination measures.

Put laundry away was an item on the list, but then it ballooned into *Shit. The entire drawer is a mess.*

That meant that, when I finished the laundry, I would have to pull everything out of all the drawers and reorganize them because they weren't how they should be.

Bottom line: While she solved the physical clutter, she didn't exactly clear out the mental clutter.

No Is an Answer, Too

The two best pieces of advice I ever received as an adult (that weren't from my parents) came from my friend Sherri. Not a healer or a self-help guru or a shrink, rather an insightful friend.

When I was stressed out that my agent or someone didn't call me back, or something went wrong at work and I internalized it as my fault, Sherri once said: *Not everything is about you.* Genius. Those words changed my life.

More critically, Sherri noticed my inability to say no to things and once said, "No is an answer, too." Ultra. Genius. Though it took me a long time to say no as often as it needed to be said.

But saying no grew more doable for me post-Marie Kondo. Suddenly programmed to decide whether my torn leather jacket still brought me joy, I started to apply the same measure to life in general.

*If it brings me joy...*what an interesting concept.

Did the world open up for me once I had nothing to wear? Maybe, maybe not. We'll never be able to measure if my successes were due to my empty closets.

But, even though Marie Kondo didn't prescribe it, I started applying the joy measure to almost everything else I did in my life, not just what I owned. I started assessing actions by how much joy they brought me. In doing so, I began to notice that I did a lot of things that I didn't feel like doing and that caused me stress.

Perhaps some people already *only* did things that brought them joy. I have never been one of those people. Hurting people's feelings is a thing I hate to do—I'm extra cautious about it, maybe because mine are easily hurt.

Since I'm sensitive, saying no is generally challenging for me, even for the seemingly innocuous situations that shouldn't upset someone. Rarely will you hear me simply say no to a request. There will be some hemming and hawing and explaining. I'll often say, "Well, maybe" instead. My friend Sandra said that that is Canadian for "No."

Translation: I am easily convinced to do things I have no interest in doing. I can get backed into a plan that I don't particularly want to participate in and frequently get stuck, unable to find a way out. A lot. Partly out of obligation and partly out of some distorted empathy, of not wanting to make someone feel bad by not participating.

My Rainbow Healer described my "yes" habit in a different way.

She said I had a fear of not being liked, based on some traumatic incidents that must have occurred in my life. Three, specifically, according to her—one each at varying stages in life, starting from when we were all young.

So I had to think about that. I didn't have a traumatic childhood. In fact, it was anything but.

But since I was embracing the notion of healing with rainbows, I dug deep and came up with two things that stuck with me, with an apology to anyone who has suffered a truly traumatic experience in their life. By comparison, these are quite mild.

Theoretically Traumatic Situation 1: When I was three or four, my grandma (my mom's mom, Mary) was babysitting me. Why it was just me and no siblings were around, I have no clue. Where everybody was, I have no clue. But there I was.

I was outside on a sunny spring day, playing with some neighborhood kids. At some point, the decision was made that we were all done playing. So I went into the backyard of my house, sat on the round, dark gray slate coffee-height table on the patio, and stared through the gate to the street. Not for any good reason. That's simply where I sat, in my stretchy navy polyester pants with seams down the front of the legs.

As I stared through the gate, I suddenly noticed the kids were back out playing again, almost as if they had sent me home intentionally to shake me, and then reemerged after they'd gotten rid of me. That hurt my feelings.

What did I do? I didn't go out and demand an answer. I did not assume they were passing back by to get to their homes. I didn't even cry. No, I sat there and watched them play without me, but I was distraught. I pooped in my pants.

That's not exactly how I'd handle that situation today, and I can state unequivocally that that was my one and only pants-pooping situation post-diapers. But that's what I did.

The poop wasn't the trauma, but the dismissal perhaps was, though I feel like there are a lot of dots to connect between me agreeing to drive someone I barely know to the train station on a sunny beach day and some kids ending a play day early when I was four. But that was as much trauma as I was consciously aware of at that stage.

Theoretically Traumatic Situation 2: There was one incident in grade eight (we say grade eight in Canada, not eighth grade, and while I've stopped saying "eh" anywhere but at home with my family, along with out and about, sorry, I can't shake the grade situation) when some girlfriends all ganged up and pulled my bra off me. I wasn't exposed or anything like that, but they pulled it from under my shirt, and, as I write this, there's no way for me to describe why or what the circumstances surrounding it could possibly have been, but they were laughing. I felt humiliated, but I pretended I didn't by laughing too. They were friends. We were outside, on the narrow grassy space between two houses, and I was new to boobs and bras and that was a thing worth making fun of back then, I guess. Boobs were sticky territory. I vividly remember the first girl to have big boobs; I won't say her name, but I know it. Having them in grade six was traumatic for her, I'm sure, and shock and awe for everyone else. For me, I recall being upset by the situation involving my boobs, but still I remained friends with these people afterward.

Enough impact on me to validate the "yes" theory? Maybe.

Theoretically Traumatic Situation 3: No clue, though I'm sure there are many that I don't recall.

I suppose the fact that I remember both incidents so vividly gives credence to what the Rainbow Healer told me. Did that incident ignite my desperate need to be liked, like she said? Were there other situations that made me feel I needed to go out to dinner with random people I didn't want to spend time with because I wasn't quick enough on my feet to come up with a good excuse to get out of it?

Still, after my Marie Kondo experience, I started thinking about the joy factor and, coupling that with my "yes" habit, I realized I had a legitimate issue.

Doing favors for people took up a lot of my time. To be clear: If you need to have something done and you're concerned everyone else will say no, just ask me. I'll feel obligated to handle it. Your errands will come before my work or my errands.

This increasingly became an issue when I started working from home, because most people thought working from home meant I didn't actually work. Not that I'd go to anybody's law firm in the middle of their workday and ask them to leave to pick up my dry cleaning. But since writing wasn't work, the favors often poured in.

So, the request to "sit at my house while a few repairmen come by" wasn't a one-off. Letting someone else's dog out here and there became akin to a part-time job. The pick-up or drop-off of humans or items grew overwhelming. And strange requests like, "Can you turn on my AC before I arrive so my house is cold when I get there?" while absurd, were fully executed by me. When I was in the Hamptons in the off-season, I was the de facto Hamptons superintendent.

Another very random person with whom I'd had a drink literally once, and who I only knew through other people, was so buried in a new job that she left me blank checks and had me draw plans for her house on graph paper (FYI: I'm not a builder, nor am I an architect), and stand in line, not once, but twice, to get her house permitted by Town Hall. I did it out of some single-girl sense of obligation and the notion that maybe, one day, I would be this desperate and someone would help me. The entire time I was doing the favor, however, I thought my head was going to explode. I wanted to punch myself in the face for being so dumb.

It was dumb and a good indication that I had to stop being available at the expense of my own time.

Before I could change universally and widely, I found success on a more micro level. I started examining my food choices. They had to be joy-filled or I passed on them. For example, did a generic store-bought chocolate bar spark joy? Not really. It entertained me, or filled time, or filled me up. But a single Ferrero Roche, crunchy on the outside, but gooey on the inside, dripping with hazelnut-chocolate sauce—that brought me real joy.

On occasion, a really good glass of red cabernet or Bordeaux (okay, okay, more than on occasion; okay, a bottle) brought me joy. But a glass of house red at a Chinese restaurant, in fact, brought zero joy into my life.

The Marie Kondo joy-o-meter became a calorie counter.

And then, powered by small successes, as Dr. Ramani had promised, it really hit me on an important level. Where I failed at saying no to favors, I started to consider my social and work time as sacred, and then I was able to rein it in.

No more out-of-obligation plans. Time was tight, time was money, and most importantly, time was valuable.

Here's one example: When you're a single woman with lumpy income (you work for yourself), you have a system for everything. I'm not alone in this thinking. Other women who work for themselves have a system as well. For some, it involves selling items on Poshmark to keep fashion fresh and the bank account fresher. For others, it's living in a rental but owning a property that generates rental income, making them a landlord who is building equity and future retirement income.

For a period of time prior to buying a house, my system involved renting a house for the summer to escape the city heat. That meant that I could work there for July and August, which allowed me to take advantage of not having to report to an office every day and max out the joy of working for myself. But as part of that system, I had to rent out my apartment in the city to students each summer to generate the needed beach money. That meant I had to share the summer rental, which was fortunately with Sherri (who was quiet and working during the day as well). That was the system. It was, at the time, a tight squeeze to make a summer away happen. But we both did the same thing with our respective apartments and we both made it work.

That rental was a beautiful home, owned by two extremely nice people. My interaction with them over the course of four summers amounted to a few emails, a winter negotiation, and some check-writing correspondence. Maybe a hello at the beginning of the summer or a goodbye at the end, rarely both. This house, situated on a quiet, private driveway on a harbor with a few other houses surrounding it, had an outdoor deck where I'd sit on what we called *space chairs* that we had purchased for summer use. They were lounge chairs on hinges that tilted back and forth.

Mount and dismount were always a great challenge, but once in and tilted, life was good.

Perched in a space chair, I'd read a lot. One summer, long before the iPhone consumed the bulk of my spare time and I lost the ability to concentrate, I read eleven books in sixty days. I'd sit in that space chair and read while I ate my breakfast, comprised of coffee and cereal with blueberries and almonds. There was a farm stand across the street, and at six in the morning they'd have music playing while they set up for the day. I had heard that other neighbors hated that early-morning music. But I loved it. I loved it playing faintly in the background while I started my summer days reading and caffeinating. The sprinklers around the porch would turn on while I was out there and shut off before I finished my morning sunrise ritual. It was joyful.

As I sat there each day for sixty or so of them, I'd stare through the hydrangea at the somewhat ugly house across the street—a cedar saltbox with a misaligned slab paved driveway, which stood out as an oddity on the stone-and-dirt road that led to it. There were few trees, no landscaping, and not much pizazz to this saltbox, which was perhaps why it sat there for sale. I had no idea at the time I was staring at my future Zen, my future sanctuary. I also had no idea there would be some speed bumps before that ugly house gave me peace.

Nobody came to buy it. Until randomly, almost a year later, without thinking much about it, I did. When I found myself leaving New York after selling the Harlem home on a whim, I accidentally moved full-time to the hamlet of Springs in New York, on the south fork on Long Island, almost as far east as you could go.

The landlords were of course disappointed that we wouldn't be renting for future summers. We had been good tenants, but they seemed happy that I would be a neighbor.

I was happy to have neighbors I knew after all the infighting in Harlem.

At the same time, I'd moved from New York, where it was entirely possible to live in complete anonymity. I liked that. In Casa Loco, we had a strict code of calling or texting before knocking on someone's door, and we respected each other's privacy and personal space.

Also, since I'd finally found a home that felt calm and peaceful, where I was less stressed, I was enjoying the serenity of it all, getting used to the quiet, and finding the solitude both pleasant and good for work.

Most of my friends arrived at their Hamptons homes on weekends, especially as the weather warmed, and then during the summer it was full-on social interaction, so when I was home during the week on my own, I wanted to enjoy being home. And I was selective about using my time to socialize during the week.

About a month into my time at the new house, I got an invitation from my former landlords for a drink. I obliged, had a glass of wine and some snacks, and left. It was lovely. Then, a couple of weeks later, a dinner invitation arrived, which I accepted. At that point, I figured once a year I'd have a meal with these folks, leaving me my alone time in my house, and time for my friends and work.

But things got a little stressful. From there, the invites to get together started coming in with increasing regularity, and for some reason it overwhelmed me. I'd just moved from a place that had overwhelmed me.

Spending time with these neighbors wasn't awful, but it didn't spark joy. It wasn't them; rather it was my desire to start a new pattern in life, and that meant some quiet time in my home. It had to become my sanctuary.

And, as I thought about all the clothing I'd tossed, I thought about my home situation, and quickly these invites began to feel like too much attention. More than I wanted. Apparently, I didn't want to be liked. They were unknowingly creeping into my quiet time and, as such, a much deeper level of familiarity with one another gave them the impression that our time together should be extensive.

Sometimes I'd pull into my driveway, and, before I could gather my things, one of them would be standing there with an invite to join them for dinner or a drink or a sunset. I always apologized profusely and blamed work for my inability to join. But they were right back there the next day or week with another offer.

One morning, caffeine- and braless, I stepped out onto my front porch to grab the beach towels that I had hung to dry the afternoon before. I had been there for two seconds when a voice said, "Good morning. We were wondering when we were going to see you." After gasping in terror from being startled, my first thought was: *What the actual fuck is happening here? What are you doing at my house at six in the morning?* My response was simply: "I don't know." It was the first time I was curt with them, and I felt badly about it.

It got to the point where I would strategically park my car behind the only bush in my driveway that gave me cover and then race into my house. I took the garbage out at night, under cover of darkness. Sometimes I would exit my car and go around the side of my house to the back door because they had a clear view of the front door.

Was it overkill on my part? Maybe. But it was survival by avoidance.

It wasn't completely their fault. The Rainbow Healer had said I'd lost my voice. I knew I wanted to explain to my neighbors that I wanted solitude and quiet in my new home after seven years of chaos and action in Harlem, but I didn't quite know how.

Evasion techniques seemed easier.

Things reached a crescendo when excuses stopped working. In fact, it only escalated the situation. Once I got a call from them inviting me for dinner. I didn't answer. Then I got a text inviting me for dinner. Then they came right to the front door to knock, which, short of diving out a window and fleeing to escape them, left me trapped.

"I called you and texted to see if you wanted to have dinner tonight," one of them said at the door during my workday.

"I know. I'm sorry, I can't, I'm working. I don't have time," I said.

"How about a glass of wine, then?" he said.

"I can't," I said.

"How about half a glass of wine?" he said.

Right then, I channeled Marie Kondo and Sherri's "No is an answer too" and I simply said, "No, thanks."

And "No, thanks" became my go-to answer. No thanks. No explanation. No thanks.

I bring this story up because I viewed this as a small-ticket item to tackle and work on my saying-no skills.

And so, on one such occasion, after I had declined approximately and specifically fifty-seven invitations (I counted the mounting evidence in my text stream), it was time to be kind to them by finding my voice and telling them more than just "No."

It was time to shoot the horse.

Text: *We'd like to have a dinner sometime in October. Before we invite anybody else, when are you free?*

Text: *I wish I could join, but honestly, I don't have the bandwidth to socialize with you both. I'm so sorry.*

Text: *Are you mad at us?*

Text: *I'm not mad at all, but it is getting uncomfortable declining the increasingly frequent invitations.*

It was all so un-Canadian, but so very New York. And, as hard as it made walking into my home, the weight of it was lifted immediately. I was lighter just having sent the text. Marie Kondo said I would feel lighter when I tossed my white linen jacket that I never really enjoyed wearing. That did make me feel lighter. But this made me feel downright feathery.

Suddenly, no wasn't simply an answer; it was a life preserver.

Did it create an awkward walk down the street to watch the sun set over the harbor? Sure, but only briefly. They were extremely gracious and, eventually, it became nice to see them at the water and to say hello and catch up. I dealt with my stress issues, and their burden of wondering why I was always saying no was likely lifted.

And examining this particular situation gave me the oomph to say no to the larger-ticket items that caused me stress.

It made me realize something else, too: My neighbors weren't the cause of the stress; anxiety in general was choking me. And when anxiety chokes you, you can't always see the cause immediately. That had to be fixed.

And that's my Kondo takeaway: I'm glad she empowered me to toss those ugly Bally boots I bought in Ireland because they were a good price (but looked ridiculous). But I'm also glad she empowered me to start to decline all the things that didn't spark joy in my life and to spend more time on the ones that did.

Also, she helped me drill down on the root cause of my anxiety, and to see more clearly what was causing it. One shot-in-the-dark theory: my age. Pre-menopause and hormones had snuck up on me, and that made me feel anxious. Finally figuring that out was an enormous relief.

Not having a steady paycheck, even though I earned a steady and decent income, grew into a new type of anxiety. And don't get me started about the anxiety of taking care of a house versus an apartment (I got shingles putting in a simple patio). Considering the pressure I used to be under in my TV news days, I should have been able to manage it all better.

In Marie Kondo I had found a self-help win. Not the obvious one, as stated in the book, but the sidebar spillover of one that made me stop and think, and profoundly changed my life.

NEVER JUDGE A CLAIRVOYANT BY THE LAMPSHADE ON HER HEAD

certainty

One spring in LA, my friend Martha told me about a clairvoyant named Mandy that I must absolutely go and see. Some amazing professional success had emerged after some of Martha's friends had seen this healer.

With scientific evidence like that, I said: *Book it.*

While nothing had really materialized from the wisdom of the Dove to date, I still found psychics strangely comforting. And at the very least, real or not, inspiring enough to keep me striving. For what, I truly wasn't sure.

Feeling somewhat settled in other aspects of my life, I did feel that my career was going okay, but certainly not soaring. On some level, with that need for certainty, fueled by the impatience of wanting to know the end of the story, I wanted this psychic to help me make my career soar by helping me figure out where to focus. My desire to see into the future was not based on having glamorous things. I just wanted to know the ending. I wanted to know where I was going, and that I was going to be *more* happy than I already was.

And yes, I feel dumb as I write that.

Tribal Headbands Forever

Martha set up two appointments for us, hers at five and mine at six. Sidebar worth mentioning here: While Martha had at one point suggested I was driving the Zen Bender train, costing her a fortune every time I came to town, it was fair to say she was an equally enthusiastic joiner, if not instigator. She was boots on the ground in Venice, after all, always had some ideas tucked away for my each of my visits, and was always game for whatever wackiness I wanted to get into. That Zen circuit kind of became our thing.

When I arrived at Mandy's, twenty minutes early (as per how I roll), at first, I was unsure what to do. I was at a house in a residential neighborhood. I wasn't sure I was at the right place because I had mostly been taking in my psychic action at the Mystic Bookstore, not a private residence.

Standing on the porch, there was another problem, too: I had to pee, badly. And I couldn't wait. Reluctantly, I decided to enter the home. Once I did, I faintly heard Martha's voice behind a closed door, which was a relief. At least I wasn't at the wrong address and breaking and entering unknowingly. I navigated my way through this stranger's home, used the bathroom, and much to my horror, realized the toilet was plugged and wouldn't flush.

Panicked, I ran. I left the bowl full to the brim and went and sat on the colorful patchwork couch in the living room.

It seemed I had breached psychic in-home protocol by not waiting outside, which prompted the psychic to suggest to Martha, as she later informed me, that someone was chasing her, or was after her, and that maybe it was me. This was prompted by Mandy hearing noise in her house (me peeing).

Martha laughed and explained that I was obsessively on time and that was more likely what she'd been vibing because I would show up early, eager for my reading. And for everything.

Martha knew me. If ever I was late, I was likely dead.

When it was finally my turn, Martha left, and I entered the reading room with Mandy. It was, what I would call, a shamble-shack of a space. It was BoHo, messy, and cluttered but light, with colorful trinkets. Mandy greeted me and asked me to sit cross-legged on a daybed that was tucked in a corner against a wall.

In her white lacy dress and white tights, she sat cross-legged as well, facing me, our knees touching.

Quietly, with her eyes closed, she got started. She asked me to put my hands out, palms up. She took one hand of mine and placed it between both of hers, one of her hands on the bottom of my hand, the other on top, rubbing my palm with her palm.

Admittedly, I felt irritated and distracted by the hand rubbing. On the germaphobe scale, I'm a six, so there was something about the palm rubbing that made me edgy. When it started to feel sweaty, I began to think this was going to be a waste of my time, mostly because I couldn't concentrate on anything but the dampness and hotness of my palm.

For ten minutes she rubbed in silence. Then she opened her eyes and said, "I might have to send you home. I can't get a reading."

If one could have a resting this-isn't-worth-my-time face, I suspect I was wearing it and sending the feeling out there at the same time. There wasn't any particular reason. I was flustered over the toilet not flushing and over the uncertainty of where I was to sit and wait. So maybe I was uncomfortable and closed-off and she knew it.

"Are you serious?" was all that I could think to say.

I felt pissed-off that I'd driven so far (almost an hour!), and perhaps because of that, I shut down more. She said she would keep trying but, if I had given her nothing to begin with, I was suddenly giving her even less to work with in the spiritual energy department. It appeared as though this had been a waste of my time.

My mind wasn't open enough and my back was getting sore sitting in this strange position.

Mandy explained that I was the single most "grounded in dirt," feet-firmly-stuck-to-the-ground person she'd ever encountered. That her job was to grab onto my spirit and float it up in the clouds with her, as if she were holding onto a balloon. Then she could get a read on things on another level, beyond the real world we were in. But with me, she couldn't get any lift. And this had never happened to her apart from once, years and years before, she said.

I just stared at her, waiting for her balloon to take off. I didn't get up. I wasn't leaving.

Suddenly she jumped up. She said she had an idea.

She walked across the room and grabbed a thin brass metal frame in the shape of a pyramid and placed it on her head. It looked like a lampshade without any fabric attached to it. It took all my energy not to leave or burst out laughing, but now I was committed to seeing this hour through because, I mean, what was happening? I had to know.

This had turned from a legit and necessary vision into my future into a circus act. Whatever it was, it was to the tune of $150. I decided at the very least I would be fully entertained, because this was charting new territory in the way-out-there department.

The lampshade, I was eventually told, was to help make friction. Or something. To unground me. And to send Mandy ballooning into the other world.

Suddenly, with the lampshade firmly balanced on the top of her head, the bottom of the frame hanging below her chin, the Lampshade Healer opened her eyes and said, "Why do you hate ketchup so much?"

"I don't know, it's so disgusting and gross; I don't even like it on the table near me." There was still an edge to my voice, of course, because I already knew very well I hated ketchup. Paying a clairvoyant for that factoid seemed a little wasteful. Still, most people like ketchup, so it was a bold leap for her to make. Truth be told, I can't even wash a dish that's covered in ketchup without cringing and sometimes even dry-heaving a little bit. I was intrigued. She knew a weird thing about me and, also, it was clear that the lampshade had done its job.

Next, she told me I had a clear and strong connection to an ancient civilization. Like the Aztecs or something like that. And she asked me if I had ever made tribal-beaded headbands.

Of course not. I hadn't. In what instance would I make tribal headbands?

It seemed so silly I could barely even respond. I stuck to "No" as my answer, and I was curt and getting back to being agitated. She asked again. She went on to, literally, ask me seven times if I was certain I had never made tribal-beaded headbands. Not knowing at this point what I did for a living, she said tribal-beaded headbands were actually my future. That my make-it-big idea was going to be my tribal-beaded headbands.

Certain this was going off the rails, and that my hating ketchup was her single hit, I listened, but continued to give up nothing. I asked no questions, and I responded with one-word answers when asked anything. The lampshade clearly working, she told me never to eat corn. (Not to skip ahead, but that night, starving, I ate popcorn. I didn't do it to defy the Lampshade, but I had forgotten that she had told me corn was suddenly on the no list for me. Instead, racing to catch a movie, but with no time to grab a salad, I ate one thing for dinner that night—just a small popcorn. I hadn't had popcorn in years. I was sick for four days with severe intestinal issues so intense I contemplated taking myself to the hospital. Weird.)

But I didn't know that was going to be the case as I sat with her and listened.

I don't recall whether the Lampshade Healer asked me if I was a writer or if she asked me what I did, but it was eventually on the table along with corn, ketchup, and tribal headbands.

She asked me to tell her about all the different things that I was working on at that time. One at a time, I listed them off to her. To each one, she shook her head, like the project was a zero, going nowhere, not my fate. This was starting to feel like things had with the numerologist and I was, frankly, getting a little insulted by this point, as I gave her approximately one dozen descriptions of all of my work.

Was the Universe trying to tell me I was in the wrong line of work altogether?

She eventually took the lampshade off her head and got up to pace the room a bit. This was good, because my legs were asleep and in agony from sitting frozen for so long. I didn't want to ask to move, since I didn't know if it would disrupt her after her balloon had finally taken flight, so I sat and suffered.

Hear What You Want to Hear

After I had exhausted my list of writing projects, she said, "It's weird, I see something you're writing starring Meryl Streep and it's going to be big." That was dumb. I hadn't ever thought of Meryl Streep in any of my projects, and I had indeed always had an actor in mind for almost any fiction I'd written.

She asked me if anything I had written made fun of a specific group of people. There was something there, actually. A screenplay I'd been toying with, and had taken a class at UCLA to write, did in fact make fun of a specific group of entitled people. I told her that, yes, I had sketched an outline of a screenplay, but it had nothing to do with Meryl Streep.

She said, "I feel like it's got a very famous person in it as the lead, but I keep getting a *Saturday Night Live* vibe."

I gasped.

She knew something that I had not revealed. There was a major *Saturday Night Live* vibe for a reason, which I won't write here in these pages as I don't want to give it away before I write it in full, but the crux of the entire screenplay was fully and utterly based on one key element to do with that show.

I gasped again. Loudly.

And suddenly, like a dam breaking, I told her the details of my project.

Later, I wondered if LA psychics could trade on clients' secrets and ideas, or if clairvoyant-client privilege was a thing. I couldn't have been the first writer to suddenly spill all the details of a screenplay I'd otherwise kept mostly to myself, but since she had finally nailed something with such insane specificity, I got excited.

And I got ungrounded and became un-shut-up-able; I told her everything. She said not only was this idea great, but it was going to be huge. That I'd be back pitching it again later, that I needed to finish it promptly. Writing it was going to make me famous, she said. As you know by now, I'd heard this before. And I'd hear it again. Strangely, I'd never really had any hope or desire for fame.

Then I gasped again, this time even louder, so much so that I actually startled my Lampshade Healer. Then I blurted what had just popped into my mind.

"Oh my God! I did make tribal-beaded headbands when I was a kid."

And I did. I did! They were made with long white beads and shorter turquoise blue ones. Light leather straps and pieces in between.

Later, after I left, I asked my mother to dig up the headband art. She sent my dad into the basement to find it and he did. I remembered how much I liked making crafts and doing art but hadn't done it in a long time. When I was young, I did a lot of it.

Once I saw the photo of my handiwork, I decided to go and buy some beads. I loaded up on a mix of glittery and flat ones. I bought string and straps to stitch my work to, and of course the tools needed for my art. I made exactly half of one headband. Mandy had suggested the headbands would be my rocket ship to success; that they would somehow be a big deal, like I'd make a career of beading.

I saw it as something else: When I started stringing my beads together, I realized how relaxing it was. That when I did, I concentrated only on the beads. Like any art-making, no iPhone was required.

I also realized that a lot of the stuff I had been doing on this Zen Bender of mine had a common theme: A lot of it was meditative in one form or another. Sound bath wasn't about the sound, it was about the meditation. Reiki and Rainbow breathing were similar as well—both calmed me down, let me drift into being present, and had similar meditative effects as, well, meditating itself. Even Kondoing the house required a certain level of zoned-out concentration.

Had Mandy truly seen into my future? If she did, she might have known I wouldn't get to finishing that screenplay any time soon. But her enthusiasm toward it inspired me enough to know that I'll finish it one day, no matter what.

And with all of this stuff, I often found the outcome I wanted or was seeking, which I think is a generally important consideration. The Dove had subtly suggested I move to Orange County to find that widower. Perhaps some people would take such drastic action. I was not those people. Sure, I'd keep my eyes open a bit more. If she had told me I would never meet a man and would die alone, I would have lost hope. Instead, I stick with hope. And that's not a bad thing. With Mandy, I would continue mapping out my screenplay. I had been looking for some insight into what would fire up my career. Maybe it was the screenplay, maybe not. But it would get me thinking creatively again, rather than only working to earn income. And that wasn't a bad thing.

Most importantly, I had been struggling to come up with a hobby for the main character in that screenplay. I knew it had to be crafty; there was a reason for that in the storyline. I had not previously known how genius it would be if tribal headbands were her ticket to financial freedom.

CHAPTER 9

NO DIET LEFT BEHIND

weight

Reluctant as I was, I had to at least consider the possibility that the thirty-one-day online meditation program Alexis wanted me to add in to my self-devised diet could work. I agreed to try it knowing that meditation might or might not make my waistline smaller. If it didn't, maybe it would help trim my iPhone use.

Either way, I was reluctantly committed.

Since I'd signed up at the last minute, I'd canceled my other self-improvement plan—a course for that evening—and instead set up my meditation corner, complete with a special pillow for the floor.

The initial meditation class started at seven o'clock that first night, although the rest would take place at six in the morning.

My diet plan had been cold turkey, but I was back to moderate drinking after the self-inflicted full-on hiatus. As such, I had already poured a glass of red wine. I figured one could meditate with wine. Nobody had told me otherwise. It was also a calming activity, so it seemed meditation and wine were actually a perfect pairing. A few minutes before I was to start, a news flash came across my phone. There was going to be a press conference live on MSNBC regarding something Trump. Ugh. I admit, all things MSNBC and Trump are a terrible obsession of mine. I watch MSNBC in the morning and at night, and if I can't sleep, I watch the reruns from the evening before. So, any legit breaking news, I wanted to watch. Could I both meditate and listen to (not watch, as my eyes would be closed) MSNBC? Not watching the news would actually stress me out, I decided. And since I was locked into the meditation class, I couldn't skip the first day.

Being an exceptional multitasker, I decided to move my meditation pillow, and my wine, out of the corner and toward the TV. I knew it was a bad way to start.

Still, I sat on my pillow, and I logged in to my daily meditation practice on my iPhone. And then I set my intention: less screen time.

I muted the meditation app so nobody else in the virtual group would be disrupted by my TV. I could hear the instructor, but they could not hear Chris Matthews. There I was, sitting on the floor. Sipping wine. Meditating. And watching MSNBC. In all honesty, I was thinking about the potato chips too, which were just out of reach on the table.

There was some sort of group discussion at the end of the meditation, but community was not my goal, so I logged off before getting drawn into a conversation. Plus, the TV was beckoning me to turn the volume back up.

I got through that meditation, but, I admit, it was a lousy first effort.

I had self-help fatigue, in retrospect. My January had been an aggressive month for dieting and fixing, so much so that my January spilled into my February. Despite my efforts, I had been on a resultless roll.

THE EATING SEASON

Let me back up to November and December before my herculean January and describe my approach to the 2017 holiday eating season. Simply put, it was: No Meal Left Behind. I was usually very careful about what I ate—no preservatives, limited starch, no sweets, and booze no more than three times a week. Well, some weeks, not that my efforts have ever shown any effect on my waistline.

But this particular eating season, I'd gotten lax on my life-on-a-diet life. Every salty snack, every cookie and piece of chocolate, every glass of wine, slice of pizza, dish of pasta, and burger in my path was consumed. Looking back, I was always on some sort of diet, so I took a break and went ahead and indulged.

It wasn't stress eating (been there, done that, seen that movie and the sequel). But I was having fun, and fun times meant food and drink. There was a lot going on socially, and I partook. Plus, I had taken on strength training, and maybe that had emboldened me. A book I'd worked on, called *Choosing the StrongPath*, was all about the medical benefits of strength training, and I was particularly struck by the notion that, as we age, the number-one reason we land in a nursing home is that we can't get up off the toilet on our own due to loss of back, ass, and leg muscle. At the urging of one of the coauthors, Fred Bartlit, I agreed to give heavy lifting a try, for research, to see if it made a difference. So, squat I did. In fairness, that made me hungrier. I lifted harder and heavier weights than I ever had in my life, and as a result, I felt strong. I hadn't lost weight…I was more fit-fat, but I was stronger than I'd ever been.

I'd been leery of lifting heavy weights for fear of getting bulky, but quickly learned that wasn't a problem. I hired an amazing trainer named Caroline to kick my ass and, frankly, the results were surprising. The scale didn't move, but I felt substantially stronger, which made me move a little more confidently—chin up. Chest out. A little kick to my step.

And it happened without me actually noticing.

One afternoon, I carried a case of wine into the house using only one hand, the case tucked under my arm. It felt so light I was actually momentarily pissed-off that the clerk at the wine store hadn't put all the bottles in the box and that I'd have to go back to check. But they had—twelve bottles of 2016 Sacha Lichine rosé. All there. It felt lighter because I was stronger.

And I'd achieved some positive measures on a cellular level, thanks to the strength training: My A1C levels (glucose), which had gotten a little elevated over the years, were down to 5.2. My doctor was thrilled with that number, a win that I attribute to all the muscle that I'd built training.

Neither should have been a free pass to eat more. I didn't think two sessions a week of balls-out strength training, two yoga classes a week, one spin class, and a lot of walking was a free pass to eat, but I didn't not think that either.

Still, there I was in late December, strong like bull, but feeling fat like cow.

My weight had slowly crept up over the last decade, I knew that. I could see it on the scale, but that December, when I bundled up to head into the city to go to a New Year's Eve party (a.k.a. the close of the eating season), I couldn't zip up my winter coat. Like, not even close. It was a down-filled crisis. This coat, by the way, was what I had in 2016 called my fat coat. I'd bought it the previous year, when my twenty other winter coats wouldn't zip up. I wasn't maintaining my peak weight. I was gaining. Steadily. And it had to stop.

The situation was clearly dire. A) It was cold. B) Coats are not cheap. C) Did I mention I was fat and getting chubbier?

Before I started washing away 2017 with bubbly that night, I came up with a plan, concocted while I ate the free bag of Utz potato chips aboard the Hampton Jitney, the bus that runs between New York City and the Hamptons.

Taking into account the fact that I knew every diet known to man and that I could cite the number of calories in just about anything from all the books I'd worked on for other people and those I had read for research, I knew I had the tools to plan the attack on my waistline.

I was a professional when it came to the Weight Watchers app. I knew Atkins, South Beach, Paleo, Autoimmune, Whole 30, you name it.

So, I thought, why do only one diet, when I could do them all at once? Throw everything at it. I would take all that I knew and use it all at once. Surely, if one diet fell short, the others would kick in and pick up the slack.

It felt no-fail.

My overstuffed brain, full of diet knowledge, would combat my overstuffed pants. I was going to throw it all at the wall to stop the gaining—taking every single tool in my dieting repertoire and arsenal and combining it into one big motherlode of new-year-new-you, leaving no room for error or omission or a slip-up.

In 2018, No Meal Left Behind would be replaced by No Diet Left Behind.

I set myself some parameters:

1. I'd do dry January, which, since it was hashtagable, was dubbed #Dryuary. Or was it #Dryanuary? Why do anything if it's not hashtagable these days?

2. I would also try to follow the latest fad of the moment: an intermittent fasting plan I'd read about, on which you eat your whole day's worth of food in an eight- to ten-hour time slot, then go fourteen to sixteen hours without eating at all (fasting hours). I learned of two people who lost a lot of weight on this plan, but I had also read about negatives, like hypoglycemia. I didn't love the idea since, when I worked out, I worked out hard. And that left me hungry, dry-heaving, and then seeing stars. The other issue that I thought might get in the way: I get up early. I stand at

the coffee maker at 6:00 a.m., watching it drip, and then I drink my single cup of coffee by like 6:02. I could skip the milk in that coffee and not start my eating clock, but that felt like a major compromise I was unwilling to make. But who ever got fat from a splash of milk? Okay, half-and-half.

3. I planned to double down on the intermittent fasting by eating à la Whole 30 in those eight hours: no dairy, no flour, no starch except sweet potato and a regular potato on workout days. One problem: There was that nagging dairy-in-coffee thing again. I couldn't give that up. So I went with more of a Half 30 or Whole 15, meaning no flour, no grains, no sugar, no alcohol, but I kept that splash of dairy.

4. Also, the Posh Pescatarian encouraged, as her name suggested, a plant-based diet rich in fish. I'd finished her book proposal the previous year and thought I'd throw that concept into the mix as well, eating seafood for half of my protein intake. And then plants and good fats, like oil, avocado, and nuts, as per the Mediterranean Diet.

5. In the book *Lose Weight Here*, the authors said you can eat more and exercise more, or eat less and exercise less, but never eat less and exercise more. So that meant intake adjustments needed to be made on workout days.

6. I, of course, started a food journal, as per the road rules of every nutritionist I'd ever paid or written for, and I planned to cross-check everything by plugging my food into the Weight Watchers app. I downloaded one additional calorie-counting app to further cross-reference so that I could hit thirty points (Weight Watchers program, since

updated to twenty-three points and unlimited chicken and veggies) and 1,250 calories each day.

7. I'd also use my measuring cups from Beachbody's twenty-one-day challenge to make sure that my portion sizes would be perfectly on mark so that, during that eight-hour eating window, I wouldn't overeat.

8. And no multi-pronged diet would be complete without probiotics. Or so said the book *GUT*.

9. As I started to realize how restrictive my list of rules was getting, I decided I needed to leave myself some flexibility with Item 1, so I enacted a safety rule for myself that stipulated that if I really needed a drink, I could have a maximum of two per week. Civilian-size pours, not professional ones like my friends and I usually consumed. One to two drinks per week would be allowed, but I would try not to use them. Willpower is, after all, finite. So I didn't want to say never, because that stressed me out. Deprivation, as I'd learned from *You Are WHY You Eat*, created inevitable benders. That had been my experience as well. But: If I didn't opt in to drink my two drinks, they didn't carry over. Meaning, not four drinks the following week if I did a week dry. #UseItOrLoseIt. If I did have a drink, that meant no starch with that meal. (From *Urban Skinny*.)

10. When I worked on *The Loving Diet*, Jessica encouraged meditation. When I listened to her wisdom years earlier, combined with other adjustments, weight loss had followed.

I had a plan. And I love a good plan. It had been a productive bus ride into the city.

New Year, New Obsessive Behavior

At the crack of dawn on January 1, I got back on the bus after a long night of cake and champagne. Upon arrival, I went to the fish market, the health-food store, the organic butcher, the chicken farm, all of it. I decided that, at least for the first two weeks of my plan, I'd lock myself inside and make zero social plans. There was no other way to do it, or at least no other way to start. I went home and soaked beans (breaking the starch-free plan for a good cause just once). I'd gotten them from my farm share because I read that, if you eat beans on January 1, you are in for a year of good luck and prosperity. Of course, later that evening, I read that eating pork was really the key to having a stellar year, but it was too late. By the time I learned that important life lesson, I was well out of my eight-hour eating window and therefore basically screwed for luck and prosperity for 2018. I felt briefly defeated and contemplated running out for bacon, but then remembered my favorite mantra: *Start where you are*. I let it go and went to sleep. At seven.

And that highlighted for me the major downside of No Diet Left Behind, specifically that eight-hour feeding time. I needed my food early, when I woke up. And I live alone. My friend who told me about her success on that plan didn't wake up until nine. She could wait to eat until ten and then finish dinner by six. Me: On day one, I found I was essentially finished shoveling it all in by three in the afternoon. By the time prime time rolled around, I was too bored to even watch *Law & Order SVU* (at least No Diet Left Behind had quickly cured me of one bad habit). Early sleep left me waking up even earlier and eating earlier and so on and so on and so on. It was a vicious cycle that never got kicked. It only got worse.

Much to my surprise, the least difficult part of my plan turned out to be skipping the red wine. I got a little twitch on the first couple of days, but otherwise it was fine. I didn't even resort to the rip cord emergency drink I'd penciled into my plan. *Not once.* Also, I was surprisingly full, minus the first time I worked out. That time I almost dropped to the ground, I was so starved. As in, I could barely function. That issue eventually worked itself out with some adjustment in the food choice and the timing of consumption on the days I went to my trainer. Bottom line: I needed a grain or a bean on those days, or I wouldn't survive the workout.

Otherwise, I was in check. All systems were go. I didn't meditate at all (not until six weeks later). I fell down on that front. But other than that, I didn't miss a beat and was certain that, by the time I stepped on the scale after week one, I would be down at least five pounds. By June, if I could keep this up, I was certain I would be emaciated-supermodel thin.

News flash after week one: I wasn't down at all. Okay, half a pound. But that was far from fair. I felt good, though. Eating clean definitely made me feel lighter.

With barely a budge on the scale, it was time to enact emergency measures. It was war.

There wasn't much more I could remove from a dietary standpoint, as I was literally doing the very best I could do, intake-wise. But I could add another fail-safe: Keto sticks—the ones you pee on that measure ketosis. Ketosis is basically shorting yourself of carbs, which makes way for your body to burn fat. That's a Stephanie-esque definition, but my understanding of it.

I'd done a radical diet, maybe a decade earlier, which required doctors' visits and peeing on those sticks to prove you were adequately starving yourself. I got B-12 shots for that diet, too. I lost a ton of weight, but I do firmly believe that my metabolism took a hit from which it never recovered. Still, those sticks don't lie. And my compulsive research revealed that the point of the fasting diet was reaching ketosis.

As a next-level weapon, every day, I peed on those things, almost hourly during week two. I learned something interesting: I dipped ever so slightly into ketosis with my plan. But, if I *only* ate chicken and fish and oil and no veggies, I hit that dark burgundy point on the pee stick—Atkins style—full-on. Eating only chicken and fish was too extreme even for me, given all the other limitations I was facing. So, while it would have been an efficient addition to my proprietary protocol, I didn't do it.

I made it through all of January on my rather ambitious and radical plan. And I didn't stop there. I went for two more weeks into February. Locking myself in, while fully unreasonable and not sustainable, didn't faze me in any emotional way. It was cold and gray outside, which on some level I love, and I'm not a person who feels lonely. Bored, sure. But not depressed, as far as what I understand depressed to be. I felt okay being in solitude for those weeks, maybe because it was a self-inflicted sentence and therefore my choice, or maybe I'm just okay sitting with myself. I'm not sure. But I was there with myself the entire time, and that was okay.

For forty-five days I consumed no flour, no fried food, no booze, no sugar, no joy...and sadly, saw almost no results. A couple of pounds, maybe, but wow, not the expected payoff.

I broke on Valentine's Day, which fortunately has a new hashtag—#GalentinesDay—so sad single women have an excuse to have fun that day, rather than hide inside their apartments and eat

Pad Thai alone. I went to dinner at my friend Jennifer's apartment and drank champagne and ate cake. (Same single-friend apartment as New Year's Eve, in case the menu sounds familiar.) Having not hit the sauce in a while, that night I couldn't drink much—one glass and I was half-lit.

The Ohm Spot

There I was, with little to show for six or so weeks of hard work. The coat: it still didn't zip up.

That's what led me to talking things through with Alexis, the acupuncturist. I was frustrated. Deservedly so. I had played my diet A-game. Flawlessly. Period. End of story. There was no room for any improvement because I had striven for and achieved diet perfection. She asked me why I would try so hard on every other front, but not meditate. Why not add that to the mix?

It was a fair point. I told Alexis about my meditation history. Years earlier, Jessica had talked to me about how even thirty seconds of meditation would have benefits. And that thirty seconds, as many times a day as one could muster, would add up to real time. She had said that whenever I could, to close my eyes and breathe in and out. Her mantra was "Bring more loving into my life." I tried it. For the period during which I worked on her book, I walked and did yoga and didn't do much dieting per se. But I meditated in thirty-second spurts. I lost some weight. I did. Jessica partly attributed my weight loss to the fact that walking acted as meditation for me, in addition to exercise, and so did yoga, and that perhaps I had unlocked something important.

But something else unbelievable happened, too.

I was sitting on my home office floor, doing my thirty-second meditation as per the book, to see how it would help and how best to help her describe it in her book.

When I finished, I did a favorite yoga pose of mine, which was lying on my back with my legs up the wall. I used to do that a lot, and I felt like it was good for multiple reasons: It helped me hit pause and take a quick break in the middle of the day that didn't involve food or TV or the iPhone (I would leave it on the desk, out of reach), it helped my back feel less tight, and I suppose, in some form, it was meditative.

(If you're getting the feeling that I try a lot of new things for a short period of time and then forget about them or am inconsistent, you're right.)

Anyway, that day, when I sort of checked back in on reality after a brief meditation and some staring at my ceiling, I started to right myself. The first thought that went through my mind was *I wish I could write like David Carr*, the *Media Equation* columnist for the *New York Times*. It was a super random thought, that's for sure. But that's what I thought: how much I loved reading his work.

When I got up and grabbed my phone (why let the calm sink in?), I learned that he had just died that afternoon.

As these words shoot from my fingers onto the keyboard and onto this page, I realize that I might sound like a lunatic, but I weirdly believe I had a psychic moment. Cuckoo, I know. I'm ashamed to even say that out loud. But that story is 100 percent true.

Okay, so back to my over-the-top, some say rock bottom, self-improvement bender du jour... Alexis had registered to do a thirty-one-day meditation class. As she put little needles in my ears and shoulders, she pushed me to sign up for the meditation class as well.

Despite my David Carr moment, I just didn't feel like it. At all. Sometimes, when I tried to meditate, I felt like I was wasting a lot of time, like there were things waiting for me to get to them that I didn't want to put off any longer. This class, given how rule-oriented I was, felt like a major commitment that would leave me struggling to skip it. There were only so many hours in a day and, by the time I walked, went to yoga or the gym, got groceries, read self-help books, and then tried to squeeze in socializing, and oh, yes, work, I felt like there was no time to meditate.

Plus, it had gotten to the point where I had trouble detaching from my iPhone. Like, insert the chip in my arm so I can text or scroll through dumb things just by thinking. It's weird to say, but when I felt edgy, I flipped through the phone for distraction, which ultimately made me feel edgier—though I obviously made it through yoga class sans phone. Meditating alone, however, I could see myself slipping.

I hemmed and hawed. I made excuses. We'd had this conversation before. I got the meditating thing, obviously I'd had a moment with it. But first thing in the morning, when all I wanted to do was drink my coffee. That was my ritual. That was meditative. Wasn't it?

Alexis explained how simple it was to sign up for the course and how much of a fan she was of the woman offering the course. And that it was with a group—so it would be easier to get into. It was live every day in March at six in the morning.

"You just log in," she said.

Ha! Perfect. I couldn't do it.

"I'll be in LA for the entire month of March and I can't get up at three in the morning to meditate," I said, certain I had my out.

"It's also recorded," she said. "You can do it on your own time. Just try it. I even have a discount code."

Alas, I do love a good discount code. She had a point. I'd tried everything else. So, I signed up.

I'd butchered the March 1 class thanks to my need to watch MSNBC. But! Even though I had a seven o'clock flight to Los Angeles on March 2, I did the first three-minute meditation live before leaving for the airport. I almost missed my flight. It was the most rushed I'd ever been at an airport, ever, in twenty years as a globe-trotter. And I never, not once, in 800,000-plus miles flown, had almost missed a flight. So that was calming.

The month-long meditation course and the concept of meditation in general, admittedly, had its moments. I liked the meditation lady's voice. It was soothing. Some days, she just ohm'ed, and that was enough. And the sound of the gong she rang to open and close the practice was magical to me.

A folded towel beneath an extra bed pillow, along with a tiny candle, became my little meditation corner in my Venice bungalow rental. Even though I was trying to kick the habit of reaching for my phone when I woke up, I had to reach for it to play that day's meditation. That irked me, but I got over it by being diligent about not turning on a light or looking at anything else on the phone.

My coffee habit was a sticking point and not easy to shake. I did meditate before caffeinating; however, my routine on half the days included wandering into the kitchen in the dark and flicking the switch on the coffeemaker before feeling my way back to my meditation corner. I never drank my coffee before meditating, though I later learned I could have.

During this month, there was one profoundly strange experience that happened approximately fifteen days into the program. One morning, I got really into a meditation, mostly because of the meditation coach's words on that day. The prompt she suggested was to send some good thoughts to someone I knew in need.

Next, the coach said, send them to someone I had some issues with.

Then, someone I had just met. The first person that popped into my mind on the just-met front was a guy I had sat next to two nights earlier, at an Oscar party at someone's house. He spoke to me, which was basically enough to make me interested in him. So, sitting there, back in my meditation corner, cross-legged in the dark, he immediately popped into my head. Just then, I ever so slightly opened my eyes—barely. And I don't know if I got motion-sick, or if the guy I thought of was a serial killer, or if I was just coughing up an emotional hairball, but I started dry-heaving so fiercely I had to crawl back to the bed and lie down, wrapped in my puffy white duvet. I kept the meditation recording going, but I needed time to collect myself. It was a strangely violent reaction. I emailed the meditation coach later that day, who said it could have been one of many things, but likely, I'd just "dislodged some emotional gunk" and that meant that the meditation was working.

I pretty much stuck to the thirty-one days of the course. There were no more gunky moments. I surprised myself by getting right into the sessions that offered up five to ten minutes of meditation. In fact, I got lost in that time. I could even get behind twelve or fifteen minutes of meditation. But, as I started to see in the program outline that, in the final days, twenty minutes were coming up—twenty minutes awake without coffee—I began to get a little anxious. All I could think was that twenty minutes could be spent doing so many other things. And then I would get myself stressed out. I would still turn on the meditation each morning but infrequently made it through. I would do as much as I could, and then my mind would turn to coffee or work or my chance to take a walk before my workday needed to start. And I would turn off the recording.

Admittedly, meditation took the edge off. I didn't slow down or alter my eating habits, not in any documentable way. And I didn't lose weight because of it. Having said that, it seemed to have helped in other, secondary ways: The many deadlines I faced suddenly seemed less urgent. Normally, everything needed an immediate answer and held the same level of weight. It was all house-on-fire urgent. But after thirty-one days meditating, I had a clear picture of what needed to get done when and how I could schedule my time in a way I hadn't quite had the focus to do previously. I was better able to prioritize the juggling of a couple of things that were on my plate.

DIETING IS SCIENCE, NOT MAGIC

The meditation gave me clarity on many things diet-related, too: Dieting in general is deeply personal and often a no-win battle. I learned a few things with my all-in plan about the dark side of the fad diets. No one diet works for all people. Obvious statement, I realize. But I hadn't come to that conclusion previously.

But after having helped pen so many of these excellent books, I admitted that each had a nugget of wisdom that I've held and used. There was good information out there. But there was no quick fix.

Also, obviously, for me, losing weight was going to continue to be my lifelong struggle. This wasn't a six-week thing. And if my waistline wasn't going to shrink, my confidence over this issue needed to grow. It had held me back on several fronts for too long, and perhaps obsessing about it as I had with No Diet Left Behind made it all worse. Dieting using one diet was stressful. Throwing them all into one attempt was exceedingly overwhelming, and there's no losing weight while overwhelmed.

Additionally, I finally came to the conclusion that it wasn't good to have a diet buddy. When your diet buddy breaks, they encourage you to break, too. I had held fast and strong through my six weeks, but I noticed fellow January dieters had in fact encouraged a break. I noticed something else somewhat alarming, too: People don't like to watch you portion-control when they're not portion-controlling themselves. And that resulted in several "Is that all you're eating?" comments. If you have resolve, this may not seem like a big deal. But constantly having my diet announced to other people at a table grew rather tiresome and humiliating for me. Misery clearly loved company.

Nor was it always so great to talk about dieting with others. I initially thought support would help me, so I talked about my initiative. All it did was piss me off. I wasn't the only one getting a PhD in diet books. Everybody was obsessing over them. And every time I discussed my efforts, not just during this diet run, but in all my years as a professional dieter, I realized every single person had an opinion to share, and it usually involved how misguided my efforts were, even though I knew myself and my struggle much better than anyone else. With every "Celery juice helped me" comment came a little more shame and judgment. Also, the question, "Well, how much do you want to lose?" stressed me out. That was invasive. And that meant revealing my failure—how much I had gained—in a way that was stress-inducing.

And with every explanation of my legitimately herculean efforts to get the weight off came that visceral feeling that some people simply didn't believe how hard I was trying. Comments like "Well, you need to get up and do twenty jumping jacks every hour to get it off" were perhaps well-intentioned; they were also slightly insulting. They suggested that working out six days a week and meeting a flawless eating schedule weren't good enough. I also felt they suggested (and this could all be in my head) that I was lying, that perhaps I was eating donuts in the closet at two in the morning. And FYI, those comments often came from very skinny people who had not once had to lose a pound. Like the smug coupled-up people, the smug skinnies were the worst. They perhaps hadn't read the *New York Times* article on the *Biggest Loser* phenomenon that suggested our bodies work hard to keep the weight on us; that, once you gain the weight, on a cellular level, you're damaged, making it all the more difficult to turn the ship around.

It had all, also, been so exhausting. I have since read a lot about genes and cells and fat and the challenges of losing weight. There are scientific and medical reasons why people struggle with weight. That helped me. I cut myself some slack, as I had always felt ashamed that I couldn't control that situation.

I was always able to admit my shortcomings with regard to inconsistencies in diet and exercise, but when I observed my consumption compared to that of thin people, there was a certain amount of unfairness about it. I finally started, not fully, to be kinder to myself, and work less on starving and more on accepting as best I could. That was new. Rationalizations for almost anything—well, when it came to other people's problems—were easy. I could rationalize for them, when they were in the dumps, at art-form levels. But not for myself. I was not so kind to myself, but I was starting ever so slightly to see this through the prism of my battle with the bulge.

The strength training eventually helped in this department. It became a confidence booster. Despite all the eating adjustments, the most profound impact on my health and body stemmed from hitting the weights hard. Fred, and his coauthor Steven Droullard, had been right. I would eventually discover, two years into strength training with Caroline, that my body had changed dramatically—tighter, smaller—but most importantly, I felt empowered. It also left my strength constantly underestimated, which at first I found insulting, as to me that was fat-profiling me (making a judgment that I must be unfit because my waist was thick), but eventually kind of amazing, for example when I lifted a mattress, stunning an observer who had insisted I could not.

I concluded that many diets were close to the same. And they were similar to how I frequently ate anyway, when I wasn't "on a diet." Low starch, good proteins, good fats—they all had the same bones. Add to that limited sugar, healthy fats, and no preservatives. Just eating that way, like Keri Gans, author of *The Small Change Diet*, had told me often, was logical. "Just look at your plate," she would say. "Fill it half with veggies, one quarter with high-fiber carbs (quinoa and sweet potato), and one quarter with protein." She also said to add a little fat and mix up your food choices throughout the day. Boom. That would have been easier for me, if only I'd just stuck to that simple path all along.

One final nugget was forming in my head post No Diet Left Behind: Perhaps the root cause of all of my junk—dating, home, work, and more—stemmed from my frustration with my waistline.

While the scale didn't actually move in any meaningful way during No Diet Left Behind, I ate clean, I remained calm, and maybe that combined with the meditation gave me a new view on the world. It was, after all, on the tail end of this regime that I eventually had an important epiphany.

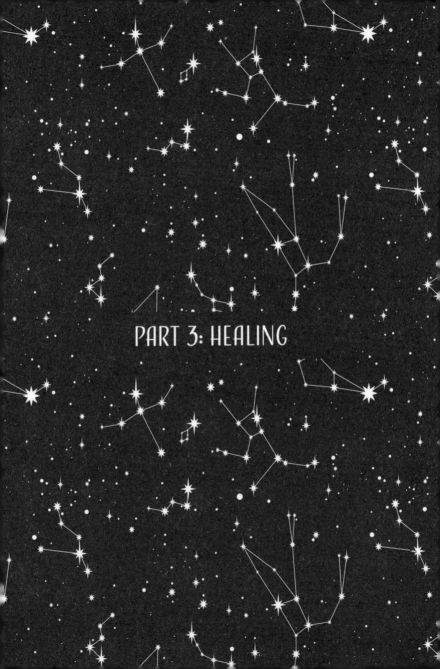

PART 3: HEALING

CHAPTER 10

WHEN A-TYPES SPA

going for it

Stunning late-life revelation: I'm built to spa.

A destination spa is full-on Wellness Central, rife with an endless menu of fixes available. As in: all-you-do-all-day-is-spa kind of spa. Maximum Zen Bender. Days-long Zen Bendering. It's really glorious and, as I learned surprisingly late, I excel at spa'ing. Considering my proclivity to all things self-improvement, I can't believe I didn't discover just how amazingly good it feels to spa until age forty-nine, when my friend Lucy invited me to join a group of super-successful and amazing women for their annual trip to Miraval Resort in Tucson, Arizona.

Hesitant at first to spend the money, I heeded the wisdom of the numerologist to not be so tight-fisted and to live a little. Spending wildly generally gave me pause. It's not in my DNA. Our house at Christmas is always decorated with these cute little Mr. and Mrs. Claus figures, crafted out of cotton and felt. My mother once told me she had to save up to buy them. They were five dollars each (back in the eighties), and she would go and drop off partial payment to the person who made them until she fully owned them. Stories like that do indeed tug at my frugal heart and mind and make me feel like an asshole for overspending. Still, I decided I needed actual days off (ask any freelancer, they don't usually exist), and I had the money in the bank to go. It sounded like what I needed at the time.

I had met a couple of the women previously, but I was introduced to the ten or so others by email in an organizational mailer that was sent approximately eight weeks before we spa'ed. There were some clear directions in this launch email (I *love* directions, both giving them and receiving them): Sign up for activities early (I love activities and I love being early), even those that are listed as free, because they fill up fast. I knew from the email that these were my kind of people—real plan-ahead types (or at least Carrie the main organizer was, for sure). And so far, planning to spa (planning anything) was something I was good at. And loved. I give good schedule.

So, plan ahead I did.

I needed to cram as much activity as humanly possible into this four-day adventure so I could truly relax. How would I be able to decompress if I felt the stress of a wasted minute while on this getaway?

Not one minute would be left to chance. Being idle, potentially missing a fix or a seminar or a coach, was not an option.

Within minutes of receiving Carrie's email, I logged into the Miraval activities calendar and started a chart (I love charts) on my computer. I made an A, B, and C list of things I ~~wanted~~ *had* to do, and then charted them out according to date and time—eliminating, adding, and shuffling—prioritizing my A-list items, highlighting in yellow the hard-to-fits and in pink the only-if-I-need-filler ones. If there were overlaps, I moved things around to exploit each available second of my time and get it all in. No self-improvement offering was left unexamined, not with Cardio Drumming, Morning Meditation, Outback Hikes, Zen Boot Camps, Energy Work, Scrubs and Rubs, and Two-Day Facials (why waste your time on a one-day one?) available for purchase.

After four and a half hours of planning, even calling the spa to find out the walk time between activities (max fifteen minutes, FYI), I was set. Of course, I was also aware that I had spent the better part of a workday not making money, thereby pushing retirement one more day or maybe week out of reach (again). But, alas, I could not help myself. So far, spa'ing had spoken to me in so many ways, including my joy of being a joiner, but also of course my obsession with fixing myself and learning, not to mention my naive notion and hope (sort of) that all this relaxing would help me put down the iPhone, even if just for a few days.

#SpaGoals

Lucy and I pre-gamed group spa'ing by arriving one day ahead of the rest of the crowd. It was breathtaking and shoulder-drop-inducing from the second we arrived. The grounds at Miraval were vast and captivating. The air was better there than anywhere else that I have ever experienced. The sky was sharp and blue. It was amazingly dry. (Stephanie + Humidity = Misery.) The cacti and plants looked like museum-quality sculptures.

To set the scene (a different scene) a little, this trip was all taking place during the Kavanaugh hearings. This is an *Important Fact Alert* to save in your brain for later. I had watched the hearings live on my phone during my plane change on the way to the spa. I felt conflicted upon arrival as to how to manage my obsession with both the news and wellness—how to balance my desire to bask in the glorious Arizona sunshine, relaxing at one of the world's most luxurious resorts, and my desire to stay in the room to watch Brian Williams and Stephanie Rhule. I won't lie: This was a bona fide dilemma for me.

Ultimately, the TV remained in the ON position even when neither Lucy nor I was in the room, so that, when either of us ducked in between relaxing sessions, we could catch up on current events and un-relax with great ease.

On day one, Lucy and I decided to do morning meditation (which I was chasing with seventy-five minutes of yoga and a cardio drumming session). We strolled on over to the meditation building and, along with about fifteen fellow morning joiners, set ourselves up in a circle with bolsters, blankets, cushions, and a seatback, ready to meditate. Speaking as objectively as I can, meditation is something almost everybody I know should consider doing daily.

My friends…well, let's just say, in general, I have very few calm or even calm-ish friends; all are wound tightly in significantly different ways for a multitude of reasons. There are worriers, obsessed types, high-voltage debaters, spitfires, and some seemingly calm but still-waters-run-deep types. But not many regular breezy types. Maybe it's a geographical issue having

CHAPTER 10

185

to do with New York City, or maybe I run with highly successful people, or perhaps it is due to the fact that I have a lot of deadline-driven media types in my orbit. That line of work is bound to torque anybody up, as is the city itself.

But you get my point: Most of them are wound on the tighter side. Highly intellectual, and always up for fun and a good laugh, Lucy near tops the tightly wound list, and I mean that in a good way. After generosity, unapologetic drive would be her main characteristic. High functioning is another strong suit of hers. Constant pursuit of distinguishing right from wrong is also a solid, fully-felt-in-her-presence trait. I say all of this with nothing but love and admiration for her successes, one tightly wound, overachieving (albeit far less successful) woman to another. I suspect she knows herself well enough to know this, as we discussed before arrival the fact that taking a meditation class and learning to chill was her number-one #SpaGoal on that trip.

Quick sidebar here: I would also guess, but can't say with any factual basis or certainty, that many people who go to a spa like Miraval, if not all of them, share some of the traits of the people I know. Tightly wound. Driven. A-types. After all, it's not an inexpensive endeavor. Spa'ing costs real money. The notion of New Age might evoke a certain vision of the flaky, somewhat earthy set but, while there are multiple activities one might consider New Age at Miraval, high functioning was still probably a thread running throughout the clientele there. Driven people who needed to unwind for professional or personal reasons.

And there was zero shame in that. It was an amazing place to get one's Zen on.

Back in the meditation room, flanked by giant glass windows filled with views of magnificent chiseled red clay hills in the distance, we all assembled. Our meditation guide sat down and asked us each to introduce ourselves, to dedicate our practice, and to set our intention. I dedicated my practice to my mother (because I like to send her all the good vibes I can in a day), and I told the group my intention was to reset for the fall after a busy and stressful summer. Lucy was next up after me, as we were sitting side by side. Leave it to Lucy to punch back at the wrongs of the world during meditation. She aphoristically dedicated her practice to Dr. Christine Blasey Ford, who had just testified in front of Congress regarding an alleged assault. It was testimony heard 'round the world. Risky, of course, for Lucy to come out swinging like that outside the safe liberal confines of Manhattan, but that's Lucy. She speaks truth and isn't one bit worried about what other people think.

But that's not the most interesting part of Lucy's introduction.

Let me back up slightly here to give you more information about Lucy. When I think of people who know basically everything about every topic, I often think of Lucy. I ask her all the time: What do you think of this or that, or what's that mean? She always knows. She's incredibly bright and accomplished, not to mention kind, and one of the most generous humans on the planet. So, when it came time for her to set an intention in meditation class, I was a little thrown by her initial response.

She said, "I'm not quite sure what that means exactly, but I guess, judging by what other people said, mine would be to *stop hating everybody.*"

Indeed, that was an actual intention, and a pretty darn good one. So, if she didn't actually know what an intention was, she quickly figured it out on her own and then proceeded to set what was certainly an honest one. A perfect intention, really.

But Lucy hadn't known exactly what setting an intention meant. And that truly surprised me.

Who—in this world of fixes and gurus and avalanches of wellness influencers and self-help books—doesn't already know what setting an intention means? Lucy. Because, while I and the rest of us wellness overindulgers and addicts were busy setting intentions at yoga retreats and monthly meditation seminars, and after journaling and visiting the Rainbow Healer and the Dove and pulling cards from a deck of pictures while setting intention after intention after intention, Lucy had been fucking working— climbing the corporate ladder all the way to the C-Suite! At an executive-level, major, real job. And being a mother to two cuties. And being a wife. And being on committees and councils and contributing to the betterment of society in general.

All that, while I was spending my money and time setting fucking intentions. Every. Stupid. Day.

First-Degree Intent

But my exceptional ability to waste time on all sorts of things aside, I couldn't shake the fact that the intention concept was so foreign to her. Despite having set probably 18,000 intentions, I can't actually name too many of them—most of them I don't even remember, don't know if I achieved, or don't know what I intended to do, but I'm pretty sure, in most cases, I never executed. In fact, I can't think of a single intention I set, let alone one that I accomplished and that changed my life. (Unless they are stealthy, and the payoff from setting them happens without one even noticing.) I suppose sometimes my intention was to stay calm. But, alas, I'm not calm. Sometimes it was to stop using the iPhone. I can tell by that utterly offensive weekly reminder that pops up on my screen of how much time I spend staring at my phone that that intention didn't stick.

But hearing Lucy made me wonder: Who else set intentions?

I assumed everybody, except apparently Lucy. That prompted me to start calling around and asking people in my circle if they knew what it meant to set an intention. I didn't call my yoga friends, obviously. They set intentions at the top of each practice. Zero calls went out to anybody from California because I suspect the concept of setting an intention is on the driver's license test at the DMV there. Instead, I called everyone else, including professional men and women.

My findings were downright startling.

Many, many people had never set intentions. Many had never even *heard* the term. And furthermore, the answers to my question about what constituted an intention were quite fascinating:

Is that some new Millennial thing?

So, let me understand this, are you calling the people you think might be the dumbest person you know, or something? (The opposite, in fact, I explained—successful people who were too busy working and succeeding to set intentions.)

Next, I decided to check in with the wellness professionals in my life to see if I correctly understood the meaning of an intention. My acupuncturist, Alexis, said, "Setting an intention is knowing the desired destination before embarking on the journey. From the perspective of acupuncture, energy follows thought; intention is the guide that brings us to the place we wish to go."

Hmm. Was I pre-determining my destination? Should I be tweaking the way I worded my intentions? Like a life with less screen time versus breaking up with this stupid phone? Was I confusing my energy, so it wasn't following? Or did I just forget and move on to something else, like *Law & Order: SVU*?

Jessica, author of *The Loving Diet*, said, "Setting an intention is making a conscious choice about something." She told me we do it for a few reasons: A) to attempt to handle something that is uncomfortable/avert suffering; B) to bring ourselves more into alignment with something; C) to attempt to produce a different outcome than we are getting currently.

Note to self: The outcome I got was rarely different. But why?

From my brief, yet in-depth, reporting, I came up with a few theories about intentions. Maybe I had been too frivolous with mine. I had been tossing the word around so much it got watered down. Also, I set a lot of them, likely too many, and, when I set one, I quickly moved on to another one, not giving the previous one enough time to materialize.

But for that, I wasn't fully at fault. Every self-help book, every New Age activity—they all seemed to ask for intentions. We seemed to be throwing the term around so much that it eventually got distorted and expanded until it was almost meaningless.

Intentions are lovely things, but we need to set them with focus, like a target for archery, because, without anything to aim for, intentions miss the mark.

As I pondered all this, something else came to mind: What was the difference between a goal and an intention?

I didn't get an official answer from the intention experts, but I came up with some loose theories on my own. Mainly, goals were for A-types, intentions were a little more flexible—for people like me, who might be flakier and have more time on their hands to keep setting them. Or for people who wanted to avoid facing the reality of unfulfilled achievements (I was feeling unaccomplished). And, of course, for people from California.

I started asking random strangers about goals versus intentions as well. I was in line at the Comedy Cellar in New York one evening to see Michelle Wolf, comic genius and feminist icon, when I got to talking with a young woman in line named Sarah. She was reading the *New Yorker*, so I figured she was smart. She looked smart, too. I'm not sure how I went from *Do you think we'll get into this show in the standby line?* to *Can I grill you about your goals?*, but somehow I did. And I had been right to ask.

I'd struck goal gold. Sarah worked in technology, cyber fraud to be exact. (Clearly, she more than just *looked* smart.) And! Sarah set goals. She had heard of intentions, but she told me that she was more of a goal person. She had a system, too.

She told me that each quarter she made a date with herself. She would take herself out for a nice dinner, at which, in addition to changing all her passwords (which I need to do one of these days), she set her quarterly goals and assessed her past quarter's achievements. That was serious goal activity. She told me she wrote the goals on a piece of binder paper. Then she folded it up and tucked the list into the back of her Moleskine, always-lined journal, so she could refer to it when she needed to be reminded. Not only that, Sarah would occasionally post one goal on her wall, for reference, when she was feeling off-track.

Note to self: Up Your Goal Game. #BeLikeSarah

Sarah had an interesting take on my main question, too. She was, after all, basically a professional goal-setter. She felt that intentions were less judgmental and more holistic in nature, and that goals were more actionable and specific, designed to be thought through carefully. She also felt intentions might be easier to keep than goals.

That of course resonated with me. Maybe all my intention-setting was a result of my new flexible writing life, and perhaps I was taking the easy road instead of getting serious about goals. As I reflected upon this further (and for months after Lucy and I sat in meditation), I found clarity. I dug out some very old notebooks and journals (not embossed or soft-sided, but practical and goalish-looking) that I had not Marie Kondoed. I realized that I used to set very tight goals. They weren't intentions. They were direct, state-of-the-art, legit goals, like Sarah's. There were lists of professional ones and personal ones. They were super specific too, including tidy lists of places to travel to, things to try, and direct, trackable achievements—like completing the New York Marathon.

The New York Marathon was on my *goal* list for many years. Consider, of course, that I don't run. Never did, unless you count twice completing the four-mile midnight run in Central Park, drunk, like everybody else, hydrating with champagne and taking a full hour or more to finish. That wasn't a race. But for some reason, I had set that marathon goal. It looked like fun and such an accomplishment. I applied for years, and, when I finally got in, I deferred for years because, while I walked miles and miles, I hadn't started training.

Then one year, randomly and for no reason, I accepted. My confidence that day must have been flying high. Of course, I hired a coach, started charting and researching, and found I needed to know every single detail about the race. The year I was to run, the race was canceled due to Superstorm Sandy, but I ran it the next year instead. I could have skipped out on that goal, thanks to Mother Nature, but I didn't. Instead, I hired another coach and got down to it. Nervous, yes, but I was a finisher, and if it meant crawling across that line, I was going to do it. That was the goal-setter in me.

I didn't come in exactly last, but I was slow. It was a daylong affair, though of course I stopped over and over for photos and to chat with all my friends waiting for me along the way. I wasn't going to win that race, so why not have fun? Moving slowly, I remember a man passing me. He was in a wheelchair, working super hard. He had one leg and was pushing himself backwards. He flew by me. That's how slowly I moved.

Mid-race, after a particularly rough time with my IT band, I set a goal in my head: Beat Al Roker's time from the 2011 race. That goal was met. I finished in daylight. And a few thousand people finished behind me, according to the stats. Basically, I beat the people who dropped dead along the way.

But, as my acupuncturist said, I still finished ahead of everybody who didn't run. Holistic for sure. Plus, it was the greatest day ever, and an accomplishment I have often drawn upon to pull me through challenges.

The marathon, as I recall, was my last big goal. And I generated it long before I got laid off. Long before I started doubting my ability to accomplish anything. Later, post-marathon, having completed the mother of all goals, I shifted to intentions. The main giveaway: I wrote my goals-slash-intentions in a soft-sided, purple velvet journal with embossed, sparkly gold stars, and I mostly used stickers and colors and highlighters.

Which made them intentions by virtue of how they were presented.

If Lucy were setting professional goals, in my mind, she was writing them in a more professional leather planner that didn't look like it belonged to a twelve-year-old girl. I later learned she does professional ones on the computer at work, but her personal ones, which aren't done with any regularity, are set in her head.

I also surmised that, since it was heartbreaking when I didn't reach a goal, it was better to set an intention because it felt more fluid and flexible. A failed intention had a softer landing. Plus, my new attachment to the Universe had changed me. It seemed I needed a less rigid inner voice calling me a failure.

Goals, I just wouldn't have been able to keep up with.

Goals, like dating, suddenly felt exhausting. Certainly, it wasn't that I had accomplished too much. Was I tired of looking at an unfulfilled list, so I decided to go the intention route to ease the burden? Were goals for the young and optimistic and intentions for the worn-out modern spinster turned Zen addict? Maybe all of the above.

Also, goals (and maybe intentions) added a lot of pressure to life. At Miraval, Carrie, the chief spa group organizer, made a great point unrelated in any way to this discussion or my curiosity about goals. She said that we were at the age where we didn't need to make a list of all of the things we *had* to do, but rather it was okay to write down or mentally make a list of all of the things we *didn't want* to do.

I loved that idea. I never want to jump out of an airplane. Zero interest. That's on my I-Never-Need-to-Do-This list. Goals and intentions might add pressure to do the opposite; only the dos make the cut. But Carrie was right. Consider the murky advice of all those books and advisors that tell you to do…*what scares you.* I don't need to be scared. Life is scary enough already.

Maybe there is middle ground somewhere, despite the onslaught of noise coming at us to set…set…set…goals.

As I say all this, I know there is still a tiny amount of goal-setting optimism left in me from the old days.

Or maybe I turned a corner without noticing.

When I built my office and Feng Shui'ed the crap out of it, as per the Feng Shui coach, I Googled the height of both an Oscar and an Emmy and then made sure my shelves had enough space between them to fit either, in case I wrote that screenplay or TV show that won.

Of course, actually writing the screenplay would have also been a good use of time.

Actions Speak Louder Than Intentions

I spent four glorious days at the spa in Arizona with some amazingly accomplished women (so much so, I'll admit, I felt like something of a slouch by comparison).

Remember the intention I set for myself that first day? To reset?

Strolling around the hilly backdrop of the grounds of Miraval was peaceful. In fact, my usually ultra-brisk, streets-of-New-York pace slowed to a full-on lollygag on day one. I sauntered from place to place, usually half in a coma, coming from a scrub or rub, hike, meditation, or delicious lunch. Some of the people who worked at the spa zipped around in golf carts. When they approached sauntering humans like me, they stopped, at some distance, to let a saunterer go on by without concerns of getting brushed too closely, being interrupted by their movement, or so that, as the saunterer, I didn't have to stop or modify my walking to let them pass me by.

I noticed it but didn't really absorb it for a couple of days, because I was in a full Miraval-induced trance. I had indeed reset. The hearings had ended. I had experimented successfully with leaving my phone in the room.

Plus, Lucy and I had both taken a private two-hundred-dollar meditation seminar at which I was given my own personal mantra. The most relaxing part of that learning was that, while I was to meditate twice a day for twenty minutes each time, my instructor told me I could make my coffee first and have it join me in my morning meditation.

But, apparently, the intentions and the meditation stuff had an expiration date.

While I had been fully in the spa zone initially, by the time my final day came around, as I packed my bag and faced the reality of air travel and work and life, my anxiety level was quickly back on red: high alert. The state of spa-calm was apparently a fleeting one. I learned that fast.

Pending reality washed spa-calmness away like chalk on the driveway in the rain. Here's how I knew:

On this last day, as Lucy and I sauntered along, I saw a golf cart stop to wait for us to pass, as it had for all the previous days. I suddenly felt a little stressed.

Then I snapped.

"When those carts stop like that," I said to Lucy, "it fucking stresses me out. I feel like I have to walk faster all of a sudden. Like I'm wasting their time. It's disruptive."

Lucy at first agreed, and then she suddenly stopped and doubled over laughing.

"We are so New York," she said. "Here they are doing something nice, that we're not used to, and it's stressing us out."

"I know," I said. "But why can't they just brush by me too close and knock my cellphone out of my hand like a normal New Yorker would?"

And there it was: the crux of my spa'ing. Especially as an A-Type. And maybe especially for New York A-types, who are used to walking fast and being bumped around and existing on high alert. (Not that there's anything wrong with that.)

Maybe knowing that *unplugged* isn't my strongest existence keeps me calm; after all, I am what I am.

My wise friend Sherri informed me that in fact anxiety is an advisor, and that high alert can sometimes be a good thing in terms of energizing us into doing something or working toward a goal.

Plus, we can't be relaxed forever, or we would have to forfeit the most fabulous expenditure available to humans: the spa.

ANY DIRECT FLIGHT

aging

Writing is my widget, which means that, in order for me to make my widget day in and day out, I need a certain amount of creative energy. When I write someone else's book, they provide the content (their area of expertise, their diet, their formula for success, or their life story), but the style of their book (the way it is laid out, explained, sidebars, boxes, and wordsmithing), that's mostly on me. Producing and packaging the news was my thing for Career Number One. Producing and packaging books uses a similar muscle. I have to take a massive amount of information and figure out how best to divide it up into sections and chapters, and how to disseminate it in a way that will resonate with an audience. That's how TV news worked, too. Just in bite-size portions, not 85,000 words at once.

Usually, getting to the finish line of someone's book comes following a last-minute week (or weeks or a month) of cramming to meet a deadline. Long, often exercise-less, days that start before the sun comes up and end long after it's gone down. Extensive rewriting and staring at the glare of the monitor, back-and-forthing with the author, has often taken the wind out of me. Not while I was in it, but once I hit send and my shoulders, which had been sitting up somewhere in the vicinity of my earlobes, dropped. Then, after the adrenaline of the deadline has dissipated, simply put: I am shot.

The feeling of being creatively exhausted is indeed a real thing. My ghostwriter and writer friends have expressed this as well. That exhaustion permeates your entire existence. Anybody who has faced any deadline in any field can probably relate; physical exhaustion along with emotional exhaustion bleeds from your being. Emotional exhaustion can even cause physical exhaustion.

Sometimes, one weekend-long *Law & Order: SVU* marathon and a giant bag of sour-cream-and-onion chips will wash it away and leave me feeling fresh in the mind, albeit sodium-bloated in the body.

But, sometimes, that foggy feeling leaks into, well, all of life, and I find myself unable to be dragged out of it for a while. When that happens for me, I get stuck, big-time, and find that my long-term and short-term efforts—even with the simple tasks, never mind the ones I'm paid to complete—are utterly stymied.

After one particularly rough patch that included some grueling back-to-back books on tight deadlines (I once wrote one full book in thirty days, start to finish, and I still physically hurt from that years later), I realized I needed some help unfogging my brain.

Walking wasn't clearing my head this time, though in the past it had usually worked. Mindless TV wasn't working either. A jumpstart was needed—creative defibrillation.

A Plunger for the Mind

After some research, the only solution to having written ten self-help books in a row, with no break, seemed obvious: I needed to find a self-help book that specifically focused on creative brain blockage.

After asking around and doing some research, I learned that *The Artist's Way* seemed the right choice. Perhaps it wasn't technically in the self-help category, but decades after it was first published, it sat at number one in the Popular Psychology, Creativity & Genius category, which frankly felt like the prescription I needed to get back to work.

The book's promise was simple: It would act as Drano for the creative pipes in my head, thereby pushing through the clogs. It almost guaranteed that my creative pursuits would be fruitful, a.k.a., they'd be creatively nurturing and, in turn, I'd make tons of money.

Focus and flair would be restored. It sounded like a dream.

Professionally, things had been fine, but despite all my other efforts, life in general was just puttering along. I felt like I needed a win. I felt like a win was waiting for me and that a little boost would help.

With my eye on the prize of getting back to ass-in-chair-writing, I got aggressive about unclogging, hand-writing morning pages as directed, walking, making an artist date with myself once a week (painting pottery or going to a museum), making time for myself, and treating myself to special things. All of that was doable, though in fairness, as I really thought through what I was doing on my *Artist's Way* to a clear head, I realized that I already had a stellar track record for most of what I was being told to do.

When children aren't part of one's equation, regular visits to the spa for massages often are.

For single people living in New York, it is basically possible to indulge in a non-stop artist's date because museums and art abound every time you step out the door. You don't even have to try to find it. It's there.

As for going for a walk, well, I walked. And walked. And walked anyway, for exercise and to soothe my mind. In fact, I have a strict no-changing-trains policy. I would rather walk outside than make the switch underground. Some days, I clocked five or six or more miles on the streets of New York, without actually setting out on an actual walk. It is my mode of transport.

Having said all of that, I did get stumped on one thing in this specific effort: the part of the book that explained that I should do something wild that I had always wanted to do but hadn't done because of outside resistance (people telling me that I shouldn't).

For that, I was 100 percent out of ideas. Doing what I wanted was my thing already. My parents had asked exceptionally little of me in that regard, although, after multiple trips to Tulum for yoga retreats over the years, my mother did request I stop going there, as they were "killing Canadians." (There had been some reports of both Canadian and American tourists being killed by cartels while on vacation; my mom didn't want me to be next.) A friend asked me to go to a retreat there during the ban, which is still in place, but I told her I could not, as it was literally the only thing my safety-first mother had ever asked of me. My friend said, "So lie to your mother." I would never. I have never. Mexico to me was like gluten to most of the summer set in the Hamptons—a ridiculous life exclusion that I would avoid anyway. If I lied to my mom and became another murdered Canadian, she'd most certainly be mad at me. And that I couldn't handle.

Being not rebellious by any measure, I decided that dyeing a red streak in my hair was to be my big, wild, always-wanted-to-do thing. I was hesitant, of course. I was, after all, in my mid-forties, and a red streak felt like a very teenaged rebellion.

But I didn't want to do anything else. I had no desire, in fact, for many things that might have made sense. Tattoo, no thanks, not interested. Piercings in weird places, other than earlobes, are certainly not for me, in part because pain is just not my thing. Drugs aren't for me, not even the latest CBD phase that fancy people are embracing.

A red streak partly buried in the back of my hair so nobody could actually see it, well, that sounded downright wild. Being in Venice Beach at the time, I wandered into a salon and asked for an expert colorist, and a bright and cheery girl who curses like a sailor (like me, which is a lot of the reason I love her), named Illiana, fixed me up.

There is certainly no way to know if that red streak put me on the path to creative success, but I liked it. In fact, I kind of loved it. Being *wild* was apparently fun. Clearly, I had been missing out. It was, perhaps, as wild as I'd ever get. But I understood the rebellion of it all once I did it. And it felt dumb and fun at the same time.

That red streak was short-lived, but Illiana in my life was not. When I was back in New York for my cut and regular highlights and color, my colorist of a solid decade apparently didn't like my red streak. Without asking, he dyed it back to match the rest of my hair. He didn't understand the point of the red streak. And he took it upon himself to remove the red streak. And I took it upon myself not to return to that salon after all the years of loving the way he made every strand of my hair look. His act of discouragement was probably the reason the book suggested doing something we always wanted to do, to transcend the judgment of others. Had I asked my regular colorist to streak me, I'm certain he would have talked me out of it.

So, to give *The Artist's Way* credit on this task: Turn down the noise and just do it.

Youthfulness for Purchase

What does all this have to do with aging?

Well, for starters, gray hair.

That was the first sign of aging that I noticed. At first, just a couple, then suddenly clumps, then eventually, I needed to do my roots every eight weeks or so. After my colorist committed red-streak-o-cide on me, I found myself turning to Illiana for color that wasn't rebellious in nature, just necessary. While I found someone

A-plus in New York to work magic with the scissors (Ricky), I never found anyone as artful with the color as Illiana.

And so, a new and expensive grasp-at-youth habit formed: Flying to LA to have my hair colored at least three times a year became a thing.

Obviously, I could not get on a plane every six to eight weeks to touch up those rapidly increasing gray roots, so to save money, I started using a dye-by-mail kit for the touch-ups. Illiana gave me my recipe, I punched it in online, and voilà, dye started to arrive every other month. Each time, I would put on the gloves, pour bottle A into bottle B, and paint the inch of hair closest to my scalp. The entire system worked like a charm.

Until, one day, it did not.

One month, I opened the box of hair color and got myself set up in my finest ratty shirt. I gloved up and opened the bottles that contained the two ingredients that make medium brown. Based 100 percent on nothing, I imagined that neither bottle did anything alone, but the magic happened upon mixing. That's when medium brown became, well, medium brown. Otherwise it was just a bottle of white liquid and a bottle of canola-oil-colored liquid.

That particular day, I peeled the seal, and before I could pour the oil-looking bottle into the other one, it slipped from my hand and dropped onto my white tile bathroom floor. Startled, I hesitated and stared, then I reacted. I picked up the bottle, used some toilet paper to wipe up the spill, threw everything in the garbage—including the liquids, because I couldn't dye my hair with half the product I needed (though I considered it)—and stepped back to assess the situation. I looked at the counter, the side of the vanity, and the floor, and they were all as white as they had been before my #DyeFail began.

I exited and went on with my day, just without medium-brown roots.

Hours later, I ran upstairs again to grab something from my bedroom. One quick glance into the bathroom stopped me in my tracks. The countertop was medium brown; the side of the vanity was splashed with medium brown. The white tile squares on the floor were medium brown, and the previously white grout was fully and deeply medium brown. The toilet seat, and the side of the toilet, were heavily splashed and stained with medium brown.

While it was all horrifying, the toilet seat in particular was a problem. To be clear, it looked like someone had experienced a massive misfire of extremely explosive poop, and had tried in vain to make it to the seat, but basically couldn't and had crapped everywhere. Essentially, everything in that bathroom that day was medium brown except the roots of my hair.

And not just that day. Saving hundreds of dollars by dyeing my roots at home would one day cost me thousands in bathroom renovations to get the new and permanent brown out.

Note to self: Apparently, each bottle alone did actually have some active ingredients.

The Thrill of Looking Emotionless

It's fair to say, gray hair soon became the least of my aging worries. Eventually, I noticed it all just started to sag. My belly started to look like cake batter that was being poured and then froze mid-pour. The boobs were suddenly a little less perky than they had once been. And, worst of all, I started to notice that my face was falling. Wrinkles and jowls, two words that had not entered my brain space in my early forties, became my nemesis. Fortunately, I was already taking an anti-aging journey to the West Coast when I decided to add to my anti-aging regime the best invention next to air conditioning: Botox. Sure, LA gives good guru, but the City of Angels absolutely excels at wiping the emotion completely off your face with a little squirt in the forehead just once or twice a year.

So, while I'm certain it was never *The Artist's Way*'s intention for me to pick up some when-in-Rome habits, that was indeed the result of my efforts to unclog and unleash my creative genius.

What it certainly did unleash, as in run off the leash and out of my head, was the information I had learned in my early feminist reading from books like *The Beauty Myth* by Naomi Wolf, the kind of books I *used* to soak up before more satisfying ones like *The Secret* came along. That particular piece of literature stuck in my head for most of my younger years, but obviously drained right out the second I learned the term "elevens" and that I had them. What I had learned from Wolf's criticism about high heels as a tool used by men to keep women down, the dating coach caused to evaporate, like the elevens on my forehead, with one little injection.

More, it quickly became apparent that Botox wasn't a choice, but an imperative. It wouldn't be if all of us on the planet chose not to do it. We'd be equal in our wrinkles. As things stood, however, opting out of buying youthfulness would set me back and make me look older than all the Botoxed people of the world.

It was an anti-feminist, damned-if-you-do-damned-if-you-don't quagmire that was inevitable unless all the women of the world united and agreed to accept wrinkles, forfeit injections, and all look our actual age forever. The problem, as I started to realize, was that we trash female celebs when they overshoot on the face work, but we trash them even more when they don't do it.

We're all rotten.

And so, I get my Botox. Since I quite frankly never need to look or act my age, those beauty runs to LA became a lifetime commitment that I will never abandon as long as I'm able to make that flight.

As I got to thinking about that notion—not looking my age (not only thanks to Botox, I believe)—I made an all-out effort to tell people I was heading toward fifty. There was no shame, in my mind, of reaching that age. The response was always the same: *What? You don't look it!* Of course, that's supposed to be a good thing and, for all my insecurities, I certainly enjoyed hearing it and felt smug being told how young I looked. But it also made me wonder: What's fifty supposed to look like? For me to *not* look fifty meant people have compared me to others at fifty. It meant they have sized a woman up and essentially told her, *Don't worry, you don't look that dreadful age.* It meant we were all hating on fifty, and age in general, and being young was still the only win.

I wasn't going to stop coloring my hair and freezing my face, but I also wasn't going to be ashamed of my age. I'm proud of it. I'm not sure that means age is all about the way we wear it, more that we need to recalibrate our notion of fifty, or every age. Even with our hypocritical touch-ups.

Can I connect that line of thinking to my red streak? Maybe. Can I thank *The Artist's Way* for getting me there? Yes, I think I can. It certainly wasn't the goal when I started reading it. Plus, I feel certain the author's intention wasn't to encourage my Botox habit. And I had long since stopped doing my morning pages. Perhaps I'm a hypocrite for still grasping at looking younger, but the book made me decide that fifty wasn't going to stop me from doing anything that I'd previously felt too old to do.

The thing I was not able to square in my head: Why was I able to feel okay about aging, but not to feel okay about my appearance or whatever I was measuring as success? All I could come up with was: We all have our shit.

My friend Sandra asked me a few months before my fiftieth birthday, "What are your goals for turning fifty?"

Despite the very timely nature of her question during this writing, right as I was pondering the notion of goals and then beating myself up for having stopped setting them, I said, "I have none. I just want to be okay with it and not freak out about it like so many other people do. I want to have a party. And go on a trip. I'd like to buy myself a gift to celebrate, and I'd like someone to make me a cake."

Of course, I have had those moments of terror when I thought: I can't accomplish anything great after fifty, so why set goals? Nobody becomes a raging success at that age, do they? Or am I just getting started? I frequently Google who's-done-what-at-what-age inquiries. Van Gogh was a late bloomer. Julia Child didn't publish her first cookbook until she was fifty. Laura Ingalls Wilder published her first book at age sixty-five.

When I was working on Dr. Jen Welter's empowering book, *Play Big* (she was the first female coach of the NFL), we were trying to square away some advice she was going to write about everybody's potential to make history. My counterargument to the point she was making was that, for example, *I* would never make history. I was too old. And this was post-the Dove and the others, so perhaps I had forgotten that I was going to be famous, which would have been perhaps like making history. As Dr. Welter and I hashed out how to demonstrate her point, I kept insisting I would never make history.

Dr. Welter said, over and over, "But you might."

And then along came Elizabeth. And that made me think Dr. Welter was onto something—that we have it in us to make history.

Elizabeth is a good friend, a supremely knowledgeable wellness advocate, an all-around lovely and caring person. And she creates and reads astrological charts based on planetary placement at the moment a human was born, and she does so with great passion and focus. She did mine, and it was an amazing experience.

Elizabeth told me that, in general, I was just getting started, that my life had some purpose that would in time be revealed. I apparently have a mark to make on this planet.

Simply put, before Elizabeth explained harmonics and such to me, when I sat down for my reading, she said, "You are here on this earth to get some shit done."

And Elizabeth said it was yet to come.

The thing she told me that stuck in my head the most was a trait I shared with this guy you might have heard of named President Barack Obama. I don't think I'm Barack Obama-caliber. At. All.

But it was inspiring to hear that he and I, thanks to Pluto and Jupiter, and the 41st Harmonic, share some characteristics that tee us up for action, including being driven, and for being part of the largeness of life, comfortable on the mountaintop. To be clear, politics will never be my thing (other than obsessing over it). Elizabeth agreed that wasn't my future, but rather, some sort of significant bridge-building was.

Here's the thing about her words: Believe them or don't believe them or the concept on which they are based, but understand how motivating it was to hear them. At the very least, I dismissed my pre-determined idea that I was too useless and too old to make anything of value happen. That my time had come and gone and that I should settle into a pleasant life and do what I needed to do to get by. Not a bad thing, my life, but, somewhere in my mind, I had always marveled at the amazing drive of great people, and their desire to make the world better. And I had a desire to do it myself, but just didn't (and still don't) know how. But the wheels are, once again, turning.

I asked Elizabeth if I'd missed my chance, though. What if I had driven right past the Doing Something exit without even noticing while I was busy obsessing over MSNBC?

She said my accomplishment-to-be was unaccomplishable without all of my life experience to date. That the bridge-building would manifest later. (She used fancier words that had to do with planets and stuff, and I was mesmerized by the depth of her knowledge.)

But she said something else, too: Getting there, wherever there was, was going to take some hard work. It wasn't going to be easy and it wasn't without risk.

Dr. Welter had written about as much, as well. She had many inspirational and aspirational sayings, but one was that, "success didn't only take talent, it took fortitude." They were both right, nothing was going to be handed to me; nothing is going to be handed to any of us. And perhaps that's a problem with self-help and psychics, or rather the way many people consume them. A lot of these fixes are radical and promise big and quick change. Intentions get made fast and furiously and then drift off, unfulfilled, into the atmosphere. Users want it easy. That's not how life works.

Maybe I had spent too much time hopping from one fix to the next when a result didn't seem to pour in fast enough for my impatient mind, body, and soul. Maybe I need to focus, concentrate, and take my time.

If, in fact, at the actual *second* I was born, the pattern of the stars and the moon and the planets above set me up for success, then doesn't that mean it's at least possible and I should keep trying? Having said that, if Barack Obama and I share a planetary alignment, do we also share the I-spend-eight-hours-watching-TV planetary placement? Does he waste his days watching back-to-back episodes of *Narcos* or *Billions*, wiping out entire weekends of productivity and do-good potential?

Probably not.

Elizabeth told me that my charts made it clear that I tend to avoid stepping into my future by watching a lot of TV. I can confirm she was right on one count at least so far. And I'll try to be aware of that.

Still, I hold out hope for the rest and, in fact, it inspires me to keep on keeping on. To this day, I can't say I believe history-making is in my future, but I often think of Dr. Welter's words and Elizabeth's too, and so, I won't totally rule it out.

That's hope. That's inspiring. That's what keeps us going.

CHAPTER 12

●

THE BEGINNING OF EVERYTHING

confidence

I began to smell smoke that didn't exist about a decade after I was laid off. It didn't smell like the usual smoke smell from matches or a fire but was a sort of incense smell. That's the best way I can describe it. And it was irritating in that it was extremely distracting. The first time it happened was at about three in the morning. It woke me up. It was so overwhelming I got up and walked all over my house to see if I had left a candle burning. I hadn't.

The smell persisted, like kept-me-up-all-night-it's-so-strong smoke, that night and many more for months to follow. I assumed it was the smell of my house until I started smelling it all over the place—at the gym, at the movies, you name it. It wouldn't go away.

If you Google that particular sensation, you'll conclude that you, for sure, have a brain tumor. Logically, I felt like there had to be a better explanation. Emotionally, I was certain I had limited time left on this planet.

Why be logical when I could be an irrational catastrophizer?

FLUSH WITH FEAR

When I was maybe thirteen or fourteen, I was allowed, for the very first time, to come home to an empty house from a friend's house, meaning no parents and no babysitter. My parents had gone out somewhere and my sisters were not around. I was on my own and I was excited about it.

As per protocol, when I got home, I went around to the back of the house, which was left open for us so we didn't have to carry a key. For some reason, that seemed like a logical safety measure at the time, though looking back, it was quite flawed thinking, because it would have been easier for a burglar to enter the back door unnoticed than the front. Our backyard was out of sight, as we backed onto the Welland Canal, a waterway connecting Lake Ontario and Lake Erie. There would have been no prying neighbors to see an intruder.

We lived in a modest brown split-level house with aluminum siding. There were paint marks down the front of the taller side of the split because my dad was once painting the gutters (we call them eavestroughs in Canada) and dropped a white paintbrush down the front of the house. He touched it up with brown paint, but it wasn't exactly what you'd call a perfect match. Maybe it was a good thing. Maybe nobody wanted to rob a scarred house, so the open door didn't matter.

On the day in question, I was excitedly heading home to an easy-to-prep dinner. I had been promised that a head of washed romaine lettuce, a box of croutons, and some bottled creamy Caesar salad dressing would be there for me. That would be me *cooking* my very own first dinner alone, and I was super excited. We didn't have TV dinners growing up. I used to watch American commercials with envy—kids sitting at TV tables, peeling back foil, steamy squares of fake meat and piles of fluffy potatoes unveiled—begging my parents to buy us a frozen meal for babysitter nights. I was told those luscious tin-tray-packaged chemical meals were not sold in Canada. Literally, until this actual very second as I write this, I believed that information was true, but now, as I think of it, I was probably being duped into eating salad, the healthier choice despite the bottled ingredients.

Regardless, making my own fake Caesar salad (a major deviation from the overcooked pork chop covered in Shake and Bake, canned corn, and iceberg lettuce with white vinegar and vegetable oil that was a staple in the Krikorian household), along with some peace and quiet, sounded downright divine.

I walked in the back door and entered what we referred to as the "downstairs bathroom," situated steps from the rec room. That bathroom had an unfinished, therefore never used, shower stall (plumbing but no tiles) in it, a crawl space, unstained wood-paneled walls, a sink, a toilet, and a bifold door.

Feeling ever so slightly under the weather, but not full-blown sick, I entered the bathroom and sat down to pee, pondering whether

I was actually feeling well enough to make my meal. When I stood up to flush, I was suddenly gripped with fear as I stared into the toilet bowl.

I had peed blue. Full. On. Smurf. Blue.

Clearly, I wasn't just under the weather. I was dying. There was no other rational explanation. I didn't know much at that age, but I knew healthy people didn't pee blue.

I stared at that bowl in disbelief and remained in a panic for a few minutes, unsure of what to do. Nobody was home. I didn't want to fail at taking care of myself, or I might never be left alone again, but I didn't want to die alone either.

Hesitant to destroy the evidence of my disease, but also polite enough to know I had to flush, I hit the handle of the toilet, still shell-shocked and in a state of disbelief. To my great astonishment and great relief, the bowl refilled with blue water.

It wasn't immediately clear what was happening, so I flushed again to be safe. And there it was, blue again. I wasn't going to die after all.

Along with premade croutons and premade salad dressing, my mother had apparently discovered another modern convenience: toilet cleaning disks that made the water blue after each flush. Phew.

Not that I learned a lesson from that incident.

Re-Trusting My Gut

For my smoke situation, I saw a long list of doctors, learning all sorts of useless things along the way that had nothing to do with the smoke problem itself. My sense of smell, I learned, was fading, which was uncommon for a woman in her forties. My hearing, I was told, was also not as good as it should have been.

I was prescribed nasal sprays, allergy pills, nasal rinsing (*tres gross*) regimes, and more. Nothing helped.

Eventually, after exhausting all other potential issues as they related to smelling smoke, I made one of the many doctors I had seen send me for the brain scan. A tumor, it was clear, was the obvious answer.

Good news: I did indeed have a brain, but I did not have a tumor. Bad news: I still needed an answer and a solution.

Since no doctor seemed overly concerned about my situation, and there was no tumor, I left to go on my annual month-long trip to Venice, knowing that upon my return to New York, I needed to see a neurologist to get to the bottom of the smoke-smell situation. So, there I was in Los Angeles, at a fancy party in the Hollywood Hills, at a house with both the most impressive view of the ocean on one side, and a spectacular view of downtown and its sparkling lights on the other.

Early into the evening, I smelled smoke, but, like, real smoke. I told my friend Martha that I thought something was burning, but that I couldn't be 100 percent sure, given my issue. She confirmed that, indeed, something was burning in the kitchen. There was another woman chatting with us, someone we had just met that evening. As I often feel compelled to fill strangers in on the details of my life, I explained to this woman that I had something medical going on with my sense of smell and that I hoped the neurologist could pinpoint the issue when I got back home.

In classic LA form, she said, "You don't need to see a doctor for this. You need to see a clairvoyant. Someone from your past, maybe someone who smoked, or had something to do with smoke, is visiting you." It made sense. And we were in Los Angeles, after all, where it was legitimately fine to ignore doctors and double down on clearing passages in alternative ways. While you might get laughed off the subway platform in New York for weighing clairvoyant vs. neurologist, in LA, it was de rigueur. The New Age set is strong there, and so this suggestion was to be taken seriously.

Like all unsolicited advice given at parties by non-experts, I took this tidbit about the smoke-past-life as gospel. And since obviously I, by this time, had a clairvoyant (or six) at the ready, I booked an appointment. Tout suite. The next week, I returned to the Mystic Bookstore on Abbot Kinney Road, and in another dark little room, with another mysterious clairvoyant du jour, I learned that nobody was actually visiting me per se, but my smoke smelling was an indication of a psychic event happening around me. Over and over.

My cosmic intuition was coming to me in the smell of smoke, apparently.

Later, back at home, the neurologist did a series of tests involving my brain and eventually informed me that smelling something that is not actually there is a neurological problem. Period. His conclusion was that every time I smelled it, I was having small silent seizures.

The only fix, he said, was anti-seizure medication.

That didn't feel right to me.

For most of the decade that preceded this diagnosis, I had found myself following the advice of basically anybody, unquestioned. I had ceded power over my life to the dating coach, the Rainbow

Healer, the Dove, and even some more mainstream experts. For a smart girl, I had been pretty dumb.

Handing power over to one such expert turned out to be costly.

Within months of getting laid off, I did two responsible things, in addition to making vision boards. First, before my paycheck actually ended, knowing that having an actual paycheck showing that I had an actual job was a fleeting thing, I scrambled to refinance my apartment to take advantage of plunging interest rates. It had been on my to-do list for a long time, but in that moment it was an imperative. Second, I found a financial planner to guide me on consolidating all my 401ks and help me get myself organized as I faced a different financial future. I was overloaded with the job search and I wanted to outsource some pressure.

My new financial planner and I arranged to have an initial meeting at a Starbucks in Harlem. She was a young woman and I liked that fact. She seemed eager and helpful, and I liked that, too. I asked a lot of questions, as I do, and she answered them all. One specific question I asked pertained to how the fee structure worked when one employed a financial planner. After all, I was basically putting my money into one mutual fund (at her direction, but it made sense to me at the time). I knew enough to know that I could have done that on my own, but also thought maybe I would get some more helpful advice from an expert. That said, I still wanted to know what that would cost me. The answer, it seemed, was that she was paid a percentage of the money I made. If I made money, she did too. But I had it wrong. That was what I understood from her answer, but that wasn't the case.

For the first year or two, I couldn't add a penny to my retirement account. When I finally had enough spare change, I fed my fund, as I had been told to do by Bill Griffeth, an anchor at CNBC, on the first day I started there. He said, "If you do one thing here, make sure to put the maximum away into your retirement account directly from your paycheck." I did that then, as directed (even in 1993 I liked advice), and eventually, when I could scrape it together post-layoff, I resumed doing so.

It was difficult, though. I was still single-pumping shampoo and not going out for dinner, but with a self-help habit to feed. Most austerity measures had remained in place. But any spare change I did have went into my 401k. It wasn't much, but it was something.

Strangely, though, every time I checked my statement, it didn't seem to be getting any higher. That should have been a red flag for me, but it wasn't. I was too busy taking dating seminars. And I had replaced my gut instinct with full-on trust in the Universe and the expert's thinking. I should have known better. After all, I had made a career covering financial news. And while money might have been an intimidating topic for some people, it wasn't for me.

Years later, when my planner and I were doing a review, she suggested I upgrade my account to some special product her firm was offering. It was an array of Exchange Traded Funds (ETFs), a fund of funds essentially. The good news, she said, was that her fee was much lower.

"What's the new fee?" I asked over the phone.

She told me. It was a percentage of my total nut.

"Well, what's the current fee?" I asked.

She told me. It was a much, much higher percentage of my total nut.

I took a moment, realizing that something was not quite right. After some quick calculations, I said, "Wait, you've been collecting a fee far greater than what I've been able to save and deposit annually?"

"Yes," she said. "But I don't think that's how you should look at."

To me, there was no other way to look at it. It was, in my opinion, her job to look out for my best interests. She should have noticed what was happening, I thought. Her job was, after all, minding my money. She had failed me. But worse, I had failed myself. Her job was to manage my money. But it was my job was to trust my gut and I had failed. I had seen the numbers, and they gave me pause, but I ignored them.

The money was only one example of not trusting my gut. There were so many more. I had been focused on so much other shit—like getting a red streak in my hair—that I'd taken my eye off the ball in probably the single most important department in my life next to my health. Worse, I'd ignored that nagging feeling I had every time I checked my statement and noticed it wasn't getting larger very fast.

And that was a problem. I realized I had spent so much time listening to everybody else, and searching for solutions to non-problems, that I'd stopped listening to the person who knew me best: me.

Recently, I had dinner with my friend Alison. We were laughing about my dating-coach days and the way I had lectured her on one particular date she was going on. She'd had an OkCupid date that was taking place in the middle of a snowstorm. She was going to go despite the weather, but she was going to wear sensible footwear. I implored her to reconsider and wear high heels because the dating coach had said it was critical. We went back and forth and back and forth until she said to stop.

My response, as she told it later, was "Fine, but you are making an enormous mistake."

I trotted myself out in the heels and the shiny hair on my dates. That's what I was told to do.

That date for Alison, that was the first date with her now-husband. He didn't mind her sensible shoes.

Footwear choices weren't life and death. Unless of course Alison had slipped in the storm and cracked her head open. Cause of injury: high heels.

But anti-seizure medication, that was different altogether. Fortunately, slowly, I had begun to regain trust in myself and done some careful considering and investigating before I listened to that doctor.

I said no to his diagnosis and continued on with my own investigation. I'm not sure that, in previous years, I would have done the same.

REMOTE REIKI

I used to manage stress and anxiety so much better. When I think back to the newsroom days of getting screamed at, or where deadlines weren't down to the day but literally the second, nothing about it makes me think, "What an anxiety-filled time." I thought it was fun.

One of my all-time favorite bosses at CNBC, Tom Anthony, was usually in a good mood. But when he lost it, he lost it. One time I was boldly debating him on some issue or other. When he'd finally had enough of me, he said, and I quote, "Shut the fuck up."

I didn't, and so he whipped the opened packet of mustard he was about to put on his sandwich at me. It spilled all down my shirt and I laughed out loud. But it didn't stress me out.

Another manager used to assign me to get credentials so that we could cover various events. Occasionally, I would report back that the event organizers had said no, that there would be no press allowed in. He would frequently respond by saying, "Call them back, tell them your job is on the line and you'll be fired if you don't get in." It was never quite clear if he was serious or not, but even that didn't stress me out. A decade-plus later, I ran into him and we laughed about it. He also said, "We certainly treat young women differently now than we did back then."

One of the smartest people I worked with in news was Kevin Newman. While working on his show, I was sent to produce special network coverage for President George W. Bush's first visit to Canada, joining the local reporter and team in Halifax. Kevin would anchor from the desk at headquarters.

There were going to be protestors. As I recall, there were various places to set up a satellite truck in order to see these protestors marching, but the night before the big day, in a local bar, someone (I truly don't recall who—a stranger or an official) suggested a place that would be best for us to catch the action on camera. Over drinks, I listened to this advice and then, after consulting with my local team, we made some last-minute arrangements to park our truck in this particular spot along with *no other news outlets.* It was a risk, but taking it didn't stress me out. Though it probably should have.

The next morning, the shot set, no protestors in sight, we waited. I trusted my gut on this one decision, and while there was the usual stress of working in the news, it wasn't an all-consuming anxiety, like I would later experience in life.

Back at headquarters, the anchor, Kevin, would be breaking into network programming, throwing to our live shot and the reporter, and watching these protestors walk behind us. We had our platform built, our shot was up, and we were ready to go. Two minutes before we were supposed to go live, there were still no protestors.

My phone rang. It was Kevin from the anchor chair. That was not a phone call you generally wanted to receive one minute to air. But he wanted to know where the protestors were.

Kevin was the kind of anchor you didn't want to let down. Not that I ever wanted to let any anchor down. Or, really, anybody. But he was exceedingly sharp. I learned early to try to anticipate what questions he was inevitably going to ask about something. I used to write five down before I spoke to him on any topic and made sure I could answer them. Wouldn't you know it, he always had six. Or more. He always had a sharper focus or smarter question for me and it would piss me off over and over that I didn't have the answer or that I hadn't thought of the question on my own. So, when there were no protestors arriving in my ultra-gamble of a shot, Kevin was rightly not a happy anchor.

Here's where the naive anxiety-less-ness of the old me came into play: I was calm (on the outside) and I assured him they would be arriving. After hanging up, I said, "Fuck, fuck, fuck, fuck, fuck, we're fucked," but I didn't actually have a breakdown.

Cue the protestors, by the way. Programming was interrupted. Kevin went live. The protestors filled the shot within seconds. My gut had paid off. All was well with the world. And I didn't need therapy or Rainbow Healing or the Dove to get over it. Not then. That all came later.

During one particularly stressful period, when I was in the last gasps of forty-nine, I sought out a Reiki master, not Rainbow Reiki, a no-strange-breathing, traditional energy-moving Reiki. My healer's name was Erin. There was no chanting and no touching this time, just silence and stillness as I lay down, eyes closed, and she moved my energy around without me even noticing.

Interestingly, she found what the Lampshade Healer had found: that I was difficult to read. She told me after the session that she'd had a hard time getting in and had to work to figure out what was going on with me.

What was going on was a long list of things.

First, my mother was having surgery, and that stressed me out. It was a shoulder replacement, so not life-threatening, but old people and anesthesia isn't a comforting combination, I knew that. For whatever reason, I had a bad feeling about it. I was catastrophizing in my head—terrified surgery would go wrong long before the surgery even took place. For weeks, in yoga class, at the beginning of the practice, I would dedicate my practice in my head to my mother, and silently say, "Please don't leave me." The single most precious soul on this earth to me is Julia. If I had to choose the company of just one human for the rest of time, I would choose my mother. When I'm not with her, I miss her. As such, I feel preemptively sad for the days when she won't be around, when she won't be getting up in the middle of the night to track my flight to Tokyo or wherever, and then texting to see if I landed. I am preemptively heartbroken, knowing she won't always tell me every dumb little thing that I wrote or did was "just terrific." So, as perhaps irrational as it was to worry at this particular time, it was a stress that I faced.

Second, and less tragic by a lot, I had bought a new Volkswagen Tiguan Limited—quickly, like the Harlem apartment, with little thought. Three days and 192 miles into the new Volkswagen experience, the car dropped dead. The steering seized up while I was driving, and I had a harrowing time wheeling it to safety. That car was taken away on a flatbed, lemon laws did not kick in, and a week later, with no apology, the $26,000 bought-and-paid-for-not-leased mistake was back in my driveway, with steering.

In addition to that, my bank account got hacked, and, while they didn't get any money, it was a complete time-suck for weeks.

Finally, and I brought this one on myself, I was renovating my kitchen. Not a feel-sorry-for-me stress, I know. Please don't mistake my bringing it up for that. But I learned that I was ill-equipped for the ups and downs of this, and during the work, anxiety overwhelmed me. Plus, try doing that while you work from home. Ultimately, I went into the renovation thinking I was a breezy person, ignoring what everybody warned would be a horrible and challenging experience. I learned quickly that a life's worth of pent-up indifference about a lot of things suddenly came out in that construction project.

All small and insignificant things, save for the surgery, but put them all together and I was getting wiped off the emotional map. I was ill-equipped to handle one of these things on its own, let alone all of them together, and a result, I was choking on the anxiety. I was near catatonic from the stress. Frozen and feeling broken.

And Erin picked up on this. I would argue that she saved me from a breakdown. By the time I met Erin, I felt, not like I was trudging through mud, but like it had dried up and I was frozen there with it. I was stressed out, having not had acupuncture for months, I couldn't focus on work, and the mishaps that had plagued me, well, that left everything else clogged up, too. I couldn't sleep, not well anyway, and I couldn't shake the ever-deepening rut I felt I was in.

Reiki is weird. Initially, it feels like nothing has happened. Then you get in your bed that night and you slip into a coma. It's unexplainable magic. After one in-person session, I contracted Erin to do remote Reiki, which was, apparently, a thing.

For thirty glorious days, Erin performed daily Reiki on me from afar. She would call every couple of days to share insights and things she had seen, and we would talk through some of the things that I was experiencing.

Even if you don't believe this could be real, that I could feel relief from energy shifting in another state, believe this: There's something affirming and positive about taking a moment to think about how to be calm. It's comforting and inspiring to have an insightful, empathetic human remind you that stress is bad, and that you are strong, creative, and smart, and can get through the challenges. There's something nice about having that kind of wellness support.

That is real.

And my time with Erin was measured very clearly in hours slept and coherent words written. Undisputable, objective measures of her work.

And something else crazy happened, too.

By the time I met Erin, I had turned down the anti-seizure medicine. I had also been gripped by the worst nasal congestion and inability to breathe normally that I had ever experienced.

Eventually, I asked my general practitioner what she would do if I had a sinus infection or Lyme disease, because maybe the smoke smelling was caused by one of those things coupled with the agonizing congestion. My gut told me my brain was less involved than I had been told.

My doctor's answer was three weeks of antibiotics, which I took, and I still smelled smoke. Even more troubling, the congestion got worse. I would go to the beach each day and I grew so congested there that I had to leave. It went on for a full month or more, and I was beginning to think I was looking at my breathing for the rest of my life—that this was the way it was going to be moving forward.

One random day during my month-of-Erin, she called.

"What's going on with your sinuses?" she asked. Come. On. I hadn't told her anything about my sinus issues or my smoke issue. Yes, I said, they're making me crazy. She said she'd cleared them during Reiki.

I thought very little of that conversation that day, because the situation didn't change. They didn't clear.

A few days later, I was sitting on my couch and I was in agony. I thought, *Okay, I'm going to have post-nasal drip and green thick snot pouring out of my nose forever*. It was dreadful.

Then Erin called again.

"Your sinuses are causing you all kinds of problems, aren't they?"

"Yes!" I said. It was the understatement of the century.

She told me she knew this. That she could see it. And that she knew it wasn't just sinuses, there were other things happening as a result of that congestion. Erin told me she had cleared my sinuses, once again, and that I would get some relief soon.

I didn't think much of the latter part of her statement until a few hours later.

I hung up and, while I felt calm thanks to my month of remote Reiki, I was still resigned to never breathing normally again. About an hour later, I was suddenly and amazingly able to blow my nose fully for the first time in a long, long time. Usually, it just kept coming and wouldn't clear. Brace yourself or turn down the volume, because this next part is super gross: I gave one last big heavy blow, and from somewhere deep inside my head everything in there came out into that Kleenex, including a large black piece of something that looked to me like brain matter. (Gross, I'm sorry.)

I was certain I'd blown a piece of my brain out of my nostril.

But Jesus, Mary, and Joseph: I could suddenly breathe, for the first time in what had felt like forever.

And I have never smelled smoke again. Ever.

After my thirty days with Erin, we were doing our closing call when she explained to me that, in that last vision, she saw me under water blowing bubbles, happily, not stressed, and moving through the water with ease. I reminded her of our initial discussion: that she'd seen me jumping off a cliff into water, holding my breath, surviving for as long as I could, as it was the only option I could see. She had forgotten that was how we had started. I was wowed by how poignant it was to bookend my time with her in that way.

CHAPTER 13

●

WHEN YOUR HEALER JUMPS THE SHARK

peace

For years, I swore by the Rainbow Healer, Skype sessions and all. And maybe that was the problem—there was no take-it-with-a-grain-of-salt mentality. I blindly believed. Strange, of course, for someone who had spent a career asking questions.

I would send struggling friends her way, certain they would leave feeling better. And they did. My friend Gianpaolo went to see her and described his experience: "My body cried." That was an incredibly accurate way to explain it. The common threads among those who saw her were a rush of inexplicable tears and deep sleep the night that followed a session.

These were worthwhile benefits in my opinion, and they kept me coming back.

Then, toward my final couple of visits with her, I noticed a shift in how we worked together. Energy movement was always the reason I visited her. And she did reorganize mine when I saw her, and I always felt a little clearer and calmer when I left.

But she had also started branching out, almost as though she wanted to expand her business somehow beyond energy work. Suddenly, our sessions felt more like life coaching. And not in a good way.

In fairness, Amazon used to only sell books. Then the company began to basically rule the world. Companies need to expand and innovate. I get that.

So, apparently, do healers.

For me, in my business, the opposite is what drove my increased revenue. At first, when I started writing, I threw spaghetti at a lot of walls to see what stuck, trying various formats and all types of projects. I took on many different kinds of clients. But, ultimately, that left me scattered and stretched thin. When I made the decision to micro-focus on one particular type of writing, with a specific type of client, and to stay in my lane, I started to find my stride. And to thrive.

It wasn't just the Rainbow Healer who was trying on new hats, I noticed. Several of my go-to healers were tackling new territory. One started explaining the publishing industry to me; she started coaching me on writing. Um, that's what people pay *me* for.

The Dove was expanding, too. Right around the time of my last visit to the Rainbow Healer, the Dove had invited me to, coincidentally enough, a vision-board-making session at the glorious Soho House in Malibu. I hadn't made a vision board in a long time, nearly a decade. Harder fixes had eclipsed my vision-boarding.

The Dove, at this particular vision-board-day event, was set up in an open-air room on the ocean. It was a spectacularly sunny day. I could see how the vision board connected to her intuitive work. Her readings were encouraging, and mostly about the future. The vision board was about making that future materialize, so working on both wasn't off the mark. She hadn't suddenly started performing root canals, or anything random like that; she was still on the same road, even if she was in a new lane.

More interesting for me was my reaction to the vision-board process ten years after making my first one. Other than the size of the vision board (this one was about two by three feet), the principles were the same. *See it and you can be it.* That day, I cut and pasted and visioned as best I could, filling all my space with hundreds of pictures of things I wanted to bring into my life. But my reaction to this particular vision board was startlingly different from my first two early attempts. All the things I had pasted were similar—fancy décor, skinniness, success in some form, home, and a man—but this time, it just felt greedy.

Sitting there taking in the ocean air, watching the waves hit the sand, the sun on this open deck hot on my face, that alone felt like enough. I was, in many ways, already living my vision board.

One sunny afternoon that same week, I arrived at the Rainbow Healer's new location for what would be my final session with her. As she shuffled the Tarot cards, she asked me what I wanted to work on. As usual (almost as if I were sticking to a script), I said, "I'd like to reduce anxiety. I'd like to lose weight. And, of course, my love life." My personal and oft-inquired-about trifecta. It had become boring, even to me.

The Rainbow Healer explained that the weight and my love life were intricately linked, but that they shouldn't have been. It was weird. It didn't feel like what I was paying her to tell me. And on some level, when she next offered up, in great detail, personal examples of her own struggles with weight and men, I thought maybe we'd gotten too comfortable with each other. And that made her feel comfortable sharing her own woes.

All while I watched the clock tick away on my time.

Or, maybe she had just had it with me and could no longer fix me up using her traditional methodology.

As I sat there, I wanted only to participate in her wacky breathing technique that made me hyperventilate into a daze and have my energy shuffled around because it was supposed to be good for me. I wanted to sleep that night.

Instead, still focused on dating and weight (as if I wasn't even sitting there), she said, "Look around, ugly people have boyfriends. So do fat people." Translation: I had a mental block about dating because in my head I didn't look the part of a dateable girl (not that I'd once referred to myself as "ugly").

The pep talk she gave on the connection between my lack of relationship and my weight was weird. It felt out of bounds, considering that her core competency, as they might say in the corporate world, was moving energy. At the time, I felt irked. Looking back, perhaps she hadn't changed, but I had. I felt the dating advice was better left to the dating coaches. And in the projecting department, she'd shared the chaos that was her dating and eating life, and let's just say it didn't make the cover of *Living My Best Life* magazine either.

I wondered if she was dumping her own shit on me. It certainly seemed so. This time, I made a mental note to filter rather than soak up her words. That was a first for me.

Since that excruciatingly un-healer-like nugget alone wasn't going to convince me I was worthy of a man even though my pants didn't always zip up, she prescribed a self-help book that she insisted would clarify it all. Skeptical and annoyed, but still a loyal member of her congregation, I ordered it on Amazon right then and there.

She went on to say that I probably didn't do anything special for myself and that was holding me back. "You have to be nice to yourself sometimes. Buy yourself something special."

"Well," I said, "I just bought myself a three-hundred-dollar custom kimono at Open the Kimono on Abbot Kinney. Does that count?"

She said it sort of did, but that I needed to do things to make myself happy—really take care of myself. (I felt certain that kimono would make me very happy.) Based on nothing, she theorized that I probably wasn't getting enough joy in my life.

"Treat yourself once in a while. Have fun."

I'd encountered this before: the you-must-be-depriving-yourself-and-that's-easy-to-fix-by-getting-microdermabrasion-at-Red-Door theory.

"Here's the thing," I said. "My entire life is a treat. It's nothing but joy. Joy is, basically, abundant. I'm not exactly suffering."

I actually surprised myself with those words.

She didn't believe me.

But I did.

Still, I climbed up on the table and had my energy reorganized, just to be safe.

That's Fear Leaving You

As I was up there on the table, in black this time because I had nothing colorful to wear, I realized I was freezing cold. Shivering, in fact. I told her so and she told me I wasn't actually cold, that it was fear leaving my body.

"Fear of what?" I asked.

"Everything," she said.

"Being loved. Finding success. Everything."

By this point in my Zen Bender, nearly a decade in, I was starting to be aware of my success and feeling a little more confident in what I was doing. I knew I would never fully embrace that word, *success*, but I at least felt I was inching toward something. Plus, I could afford to pay this healer two hundred dollars per hour. I was out of the woods in terms of always panicking about surviving on my own (I'd shifted to only part-time panic), and I'd accomplished a lot over the years of running my own business.

But hey, I'd let her knock the fear out of my body and hope her translation of my vibes was accurate and that I'd wake up fearless the next day.

Instead, I woke up that night around midnight so violently sick and shivering that my only fear was death.

I suffered through my discomfort for twenty-four hours, and by the second night was so sick and/or afraid that I worried I was going to have to go to the emergency room. I made it to eight the next morning and went to urgent care instead. There, the doctor prescribed Cipro—an antidote to fear, perhaps? Or, more likely, to the infection he thought I had gotten.

Days later, recovered and out walking again on a gloriously sunny day, I got to thinking of my most recent session and what I had said to her when she'd told me to treat myself: *My entire life has been a treat.* I had always tried to be aware that even my bad days were the equivalent of other people's good days.

My struggles were real to me but, in the scheme of things, surmountable. The more I let that sink in, the more I realized that I actually did believe to my core that my life was a treat. The simple fact: I didn't suffer from a fun shortage. I hit speed bumps like everyone else, but I got through. I worked hard, but I enjoyed my work and my off-work time. And the bills always got paid. I got my hair blown out at the *Drybar* sometimes. Okay, a lot of times. Okay, too many times in a month. Okay, okay, I am a member. I ate at nice restaurants when I felt like it. I had more great friends than I had time for.

Most important, I drew the longest straw with family.

And, I didn't have a brain tumor!

I drank rosé on the beach almost every day in July and August, watching the most-velvety Hamptons sky and breathing in the salty air while the waves crashed into the sand. I laughed a lot at all of life's absurdities, and I tried not to let other people get me down. Like anybody and everybody, I suspected I had a crazy streak in me, but frankly, I was the one many of my friends called for advice and help and grounding when they were having a crisis or needed guidance or suggestions. Single deep into my forties? Yes. A desire to be thinner? Of course. But, generally, life was not so shabby.

A big revelation was forming in my head.

My walk that day was extra-long, and I eventually made my way out onto the Venice Pier. The sky was perfect, blue and clear. I was listening to the previously prescribed self-help book (I had paid for it, so why not), instead of the Pacific Ocean waves and seagulls circling, learning about eating and why everything to do with weight and body went back to how terrible one's mother had been to them.

I stopped in my tracks. Literally. Stopped dead.

And I said to the author (who probably didn't hear me): "Fuck you. My mom is awesome."

In that instant, all the intense effort I had been putting into fixing myself for the past ten years seemed…dumb.

And there it was, with the flip of a switch, a thought: *Maybe I'm good enough already. Maybe I have been all along.*

I turned the book off, pulled my earbuds out, and instead soaked up the view and my thoughts. I stopped for a while and watched the surfers riding the waves and took in the brightly colored houses that peppered the boardwalk in the distance. I let the beauty seep into me. Permeate my core.

The air was fresh and my mood was suddenly as bright as the sky. Oddly, I felt peace in that very moment and absolute clarity.

Had a single nugget from each coach and guru and book given me something to cling to? Had it brought me to that turning point on the pier? Sure. Yes—the project nature of it all, the talking things out, the ideas that made me think, yes. But, I realized, treating self-help as gospel had perhaps been misguided.

Despite all the promises and pursuits, being better wasn't what I craved; it was something else altogether. Peace. That was what I really needed. Peace with myself. Peace with my work. Peace with my life. Peace. A cease-fire between me and my urge to fix me. I'd done so much to try to fix what ultimately was probably never truly broken. I had been so consumed by finding the broken parts of my life and the explanations for them that I lost sight of the good parts. I realized, finally, that just like Dorothy with her red shoes, I had perhaps had the answers all along.

As I stood there on the pier, taking in my thoughts and the sea air, I thought back on my journey, my failures, and for the first time, my successes, and I suddenly felt like it was the beginning of everything.

Post-Traumatic Recession Disorder

Shortly after my epiphany on the pier, back in New York, I used my friend Karina's bathroom. She had Molton Brown hand soap on the sink. I gasped with joy when I saw it. I double-pumped (okay, maybe triple-pumped) and washed my hands, luxuriating in my once-favorite indulgence. *Hello, old friend. Oh, how I have missed you*, I thought.

Later, I said to her, "Wow, you still use Molton Brown soap?" She looked perplexed. I told her I loved that soap, but I didn't explain that I used to buy Molton Brown Thai Vert hand soap, too. Up until October 31, 2008.

I never bought it again after squeezing and savoring that final pumped drop out of that last bottle I owned. And it took almost a full decade before I felt comfortable ordering *New York* magazine, *Vanity Fair*, and the *New York Times* again. A full decade. But never again did I buy that soap. There's a little joy in a pump of Molton Brown at a friend's house, but to have it in my house seems a jinx—a flashback to a time I'd rather not dwell too much on.

A lot stuck with me from my recessionary measures. Single pumps are still household policy, and I'll never turn down a free razor or packet of shampoo. I finally recognize all of that behavior: It's post-traumatic recession disorder. People I have spoken to over the years who got laid off in other businesses have told me that they still feel sad about their former careers, even though they too survived. I still feel sad when I think about what might have been in a career I loved.

I committed to forever living not just within my means, but well below them, not that I was extravagant (save for the soap). I'm still as cheap as I can be. My friend Doug said I'm like a post-war German housewife, always paying cash, detesting credit, and I only buy things on sale. I wear my limited wardrobe until holes emerge. And even then, if I can cover them, I do. I still enact many of my austerity measures. I think I always will. And there's no shame in that. As per the numerologist, I splurge, but I choose my splurges carefully.

Times had changed.

But I had changed, too.

It took me until 2016 to earn even close to what I was earning on October 31, 2008. That April, after filing taxes, I bought myself a beautiful handbag to mark the occasion. It wasn't until

2017 that I earned a little more. My shoulders finally dropped, nine years later.

I own a humble but peaceful house in Springs in East Hampton, New York, and I now have a tiny apartment in New York City (tiny being the operative word) below 75th Street, rented literally a decade (to the month, almost the week actually) after I was laid off. Located where I imagined the one on my very first vision board was, but with fewer fancy pillows and less décor.

My motto going forward became "cheap and cheerful," a sentiment often implied by everyone who either enters my house or my apartment and says, "Nice, this is all you need." Break that down and it's a slightly back-handed compliment coming from people with larger homes and fancier apartments, not that anybody ever walks in anywhere and says, "This is so much more than you need."

The only person who thought the apartment was palatial was my nephew, Andrew, eight at the time he first stayed with me. Loving that I served him Doritos for breakfast, he was contemplating moving in. I said we would need a larger apartment, and he said, "No, this is good."

My friend Alison came over to my apartment just after I got it and, while I was bracing for a "This is all you need," she didn't say that. She said, "I'm impressed. You have two homes. You did it, and I'm so happy for you." I tried to receive the compliment, but that is always challenging for me. I explained that these two homes combined cost about the same amount monthly as the Harlem condo had, but she persisted in saying I had accomplished something and figured out how to make it work.

I'll put my lifestyle to date in the win jar, as a whole, but I'm not going to give the Universe the credit for it. Not all of it anyway. Working seven days a week, twelve months a year, launching a business on sweat equity and smarts alone, I'm finally owning that one all for me. Encouragement and a thread of learning from every self-help book I read or wrote, every coach or psychic who made me think, sure, it helped. Reiki, yoga, strength training, and acupuncture—you played your part.

I look back at that time and see, not just overwhelming stress, but also a kindness of strangers (actually friends and family) element to it all that wows me. Generally speaking, people are nice. Many lovely people sprung for a meal, or kept me in good wine, or did photocopying at the office for me, or made a phone call on my behalf. After my experience, I realized that job loss can happen to any of us, and so I make it a point to return the favor when asked.

And frankly, looking outward, helping other people, that's healing too. And all the wellness and soul-searching can be a cautionary tale. I became a born-again and got preachy each time I read a book or learned a regime or ate a certain way and felt great for five minutes. Spending so much time on all this stuff…fixing and fixing and fixing…makes us a self-centered set of humans.

After my epiphany, was life Easy Street? No. Life will always feel like walking through mud. That's because life is, generally, hard. It's great and messy and fun, and full of ups and downs. I don't want to detract from other people's struggles with illness or financial hardships or horrible issues—for them it's much more severe than for me. But even for those of us who have it easier, life is real work. And no psychic or guru will make it that much easier.

Happy-ish

I used to work with a woman a long time ago who, when you said, "How are you?" would always enthusiastically say "Great." Every time. And you know what I used to think? *Bullshit.* There's no way everyone can always be that great. Every. Single. Day. It's New York. Everyone has something semi-legit to complain about. And non-legit complaining is also fully encouraged and welcome.

Did she just not want to share her mess with me? Or were there people, like this woman, who always had it so great that nothing got them down?

Bottom line: We can't be happy all the time, but I think we can strive for content. That is not overshooting. Always happy is just not achievable, *and that's okay.* Plus, it's hard work and stressful to have to be so damn happy and meet the pressure of all the experts and such that push for it. And some days, we're just not our best and we're never going to be. Or maybe we actually are *our* best and we just don't see it. And that is okay too. Best is relative. If we focus on keeping our eyes on our own mat, like they always tell us to do in yoga, and don't worry about what our neighbor is doing or what our friends are earning or who they're dating, life won't always feel so heavy.

One way to do that is to find your speed. I'm working to find mine.

And I try to keep a few more notions top of mind as well:

Try a little acceptance. Ha, ha, ha, I say! I'm terrible at listening to my own advice, but I do try to remind myself that it will all be okay. I will be okay. Trauma notwithstanding, we all will.

When I told Jessica once how so many people said that losing my job would be the best thing that ever happened and asked her how I would know if it was, her response was cuttingly genius. She asked, "Why, are you keeping score?" I do like the freedom of working for myself, but I truly miss Career Number One. And I'm also okay admitting that I'm occasionally still bummed about it all. I feel fine not pretending. Yeah, hello, Instagram and Facebook, I'm talking to you. As such, I disagree with the saying, "Don't cry over spilt milk." I say, cry. Then go eat chips. Then *make a plan*.

Having said all that, I've never been a regretful person. I look forward far too much—maybe that's the producer in me. But I don't really look back. Overall, I have few regrets. I regret not getting a mouth guard when I first was told to do so by a dentist for teeth grinding (which I do even in yoga), and I fully regret that stupid Volkswagen, but honestly, that is it.

I told Dr. Ramani once that I just wanted to get to a point where I wasn't so stressed-out about everything—money, being successful, body image, worrying about aging parents and worse, worrying about not having aging parents, and worrying about dying alone.

"You're never *not* going to stress about all those things," she said. That was a long time ago, and until this writing, I had forgotten her wisdom. Own your stress. No matter what, the anxiety creeps in. That is an important realization. Anxiety came with age as the stakes of life got higher. Instead of trying to eliminate it with every wild and radical effort, I finally realized just loosening the valve on it was good enough. And knowing it when I saw it helped too.

And engage intelligent healers! Mine are super smart in so many ways, related and unrelated to their fields, that, just like my brainy friends, I learn from and am motivated by their wisdom.

Reflecting on all that I had done on my Zen Bender, I made a mental checklist of what would stay and what would go in an effort to stay calm and ease anxiety going forward: Yoga is a keeper. Acupuncture chills me out. Meditation works (I could do better on that front), and Reiki puts me to sleep. Sleep is good.

As far as the rest of it? It can't be all-consuming. There is a lot of noise out there. Pull a thread from each book you read or each coach you hire, but don't lose your ability to check your gut and participate in your own decisions and actions. Listen and filter, though, I acknowledge, the placebo effect is a real thing. If someone believes something is working for them, it sometimes makes it so. That's because the brain can be convincing. That makes the motivation and action that comes from the healer du jour a worthy piece of wisdom.

Even though I've slaughtered a lot of sacred cows (my friend Suzan's initial observation when she first read this) in these pages, that wasn't my intention. I still love it all. And there's a reason the industry for self-help and New Age has exploded. Some of these practices really work. And they can be fun.

Plus, believing is powerful. We all want to believe. And that's okay, because believing is good, like potato chips, if consumed in moderation.

Dissatisfaction is very raw and bleeds into various areas of life. One big thing I have learned from all this is that, when I was dissatisfied with one element of my life, it quickly spread. And that meant I could see a lot of holes that needed fixing. If I really whittled it down, the disorganized home, the dating struggles, the screenplays-to-be-written, the money, none of those were the real issue. Trying to knock twenty pounds off—that's what truly bugged the shit out of me all along. I'd like to say I have stopped checking the scale. I haven't. But I'm a little less hung up on it.

At least I know that I'm a work in progress and I always will be. My trainer, Caroline, tells me almost weekly that I'm very hard on myself. When I tell her that I'm frustrated that this bulge or this ripple won't go away, she asks, "Can you accept that?" I'd like to say yes, but I probably never will. But I will not take heroic measures anymore to change it.

And one more thing.

My Reiki healer Erin told me that walking is actually a chaining exercise and that it makes sense that I work through junk and clear my head when I walk. She said that walking activates the left side of the brain, which is for logic and problem-solving. Walking is a left-right-left-right movement (like running, stair climbing, and as Erin said, "Even cutting with scissors") that triggers that thinking. That's why, when I get all clogged up, I'm unclogged by the end of a walk.

Jessica told me that walking, for me, is meditative, which is why during the times when I walk and walk and walk without missing a day, I lose weight. Because I'm not freaking out, and my body is calm and my mind is still.

Walking, for me, is the single best tool in my arsenal for all of it—thinking, calming down, meditating, getting centered, feeling better about myself. That's how I process things, by putting one foot in front of the other. It's the simplest and least expensive form of self-help, too. No coach, book, or chant required. It's often when I write and figure out solutions to problems I couldn't solve at the keyboard. That doesn't mean it's enough for everybody, but it works for me.

Walking, is, and has been all along, my spiritual seeking. I just forgot for a while and started grabbing at everything else.

Now, every time I walk out on that pier, or along the beach, or at high speed through the streets of New York, I remember what my dad said, his words maybe the most important lesson of my life— that what I was born with was indeed enough.

I am finally just happy I have two arms and two legs.

The Zen Bender Anti-Self-Help Doctrine (My Antidote to Overdosing on Advice, Self-Help, and New Age Fixes)

Plant a vegetable garden or pick vegetables at a farm.

Do yoga, as much for your brain as for your body.

Chase strong, not thin.

Only stress about the actual tangible things that are happening in front of you, not all the hypotheticals swirling in your head.

Be gracious with your words; you don't have to say out loud every thought that pops into your head.

Don't compare.

Listen more than you talk.

Be generous with your time.

Take the time to receive what a friend has to offer.

Call, don't text. Especially your mom.

Know that a bad day can also be a good one.

Get a blowout. There's very little a visit to the *Drybar* can't fix. (If your pants feel snug, at least your hair will look great.)

Do acupuncture as preventive medicine, not just for an injury.

Volunteer or dedicate time to a cause that's important to you (a.k.a. stop focusing on you and focus on others).

Read *The Confidence Code*. It is life-altering.

Find a community or build a community.

Get over yourself.

ACKNOWLEDGMENTS

I crowdsource my life. I ask multiple people what they think about almost every decision or situation before settling in on my move. I like to information gather and I like to front-load my stress (pre-stressing, I call it), understanding various outcomes ahead of time. Writing this book was no exception. It took the support of my entire hive, and then some, for me to muster the oomph to put it all on the page and set it free in the book-o-sphere. A heartfelt thanks to all of my encouraging friends for listening and listening and listening, and talking through chapters at great length. But also, thank you for all the cheerleading. On the days when you think you suck (I have many), call my friends. Their confidence in me is heartwarming.

To everybody I've ever written for, edited for, and collaborated with, thank you for all that you taught me. I have learned some things, and changed some things, thanks to your wisdom. What, in many cases, started out as work evolved into cherished friendships.

Without an office full of co-workers, we writers have to form a virtual one—calling on each other for proofreads, contract issues, creative conundrums, and just general company. At no time was this more critical and needed than in the writing of this book. Chief among my virtual office mates, my Head Virtual Office Mate, is fellow writer and valued friend Sherri Rifkin, whose early reads and repeated edits, steady encouragement, pep talks, and advice were the perfect antidote for writer's stress and insecurity. Focus and finish.

And to Suzan Colon for the mother of all saves. I thank you for your wisdom and edits, your patience and prodding, and your oh-so-genius suggestion for a way to bring it all home, especially since you were generously offering up your time while you were on a writing deadline of your own. It was critical and appreciated.

And thank you both for our Wagamama Summits. They save me.

The lovely Lara Asher, whose guidance, and admission that she had multiple vision boards going at once, kept me on the right track.

Sandra Moreno, my fellow empire builder and friend, for plotting, planning, suggesting, reading, and promoting. Thank you for sparing your time and patience.

In the women-helping-women department, a sincere thanks to Lucy Fato and Karina Byrne, whose encouragement and generosity are mind-blowing. Thank you both for every kind gesture that probably felt regular and small to you but was enormous to me. I worship you both.

And to my Official Wellness Team: Alexis Arvidson and Erin Tschantret, I love your wisdom, your healing powers, your calm demeanor, and just generally spending time with each of you. And Elizabeth Dietz, thank you for reminding me to think big at a key point in time. Caroline Cashin, thanks for kicking my butt. And Lisa Zaloga, thanks for keeping me grounded. To my Unofficial Wellness Team and Chicks Who Farm, Lori Spechler and Martha McCully, for sanity checks, walks, yoga, and sharing the supreme gratification of digging potatoes from the ground or finding a rogue radicchio in the rough.

Diana Nuhn: You are magic. You make magic. I thank you for your guidance on the most important piece of the equation.

To Erik Jackson, for creative consultation and writing pep talks over dumplings. To Jennifer Wright and Samantha Wright for some painfully last-minute, frantic (albeit oceanside) edits, and a general enthusiasm for, and enormous contribution to, my work.

And, since every drop of water makes a pond, not one word I've ever written would sound right if not for all that I learned from a long list of writing teachers, especially Jennifer Belle. She, along with an A-team writing workshop made up of Kathryn Kellinger, Michael Sears, and Desiree Rhine, helped with the foundation of this book without even knowing it.

Maura Teitelbaum, my agent throughout my entire decade-long Zen Bender, I thank you. You are a shark and a sheer force.

And to my lawyer, Elizabeth Corradino, whose patience and calm demeanor keep me out of trouble. Thanks for always making time for me and answering the often tiny and sometimes dumb questions.

To Brenda Knight, Robin Miller, Natasha Vera, Hannah Jorstad Paulsen, Merritt Smail, and the entire team at Mango, thank you. Morgane Leoni: Thanks for nailing it.

Erin Turner, thanks for climbing that damn ladder on command.

To Jacqueline Krikorian, for an endless stream of support and encouragement, the occasional software purchase, and the comfort of knowing you will be there in a pinch.

To Jennifer Krikorian, for spending endless hours watching '80s music videos as we perfected our dance moves, for having a killer sense of humor ("What's your second favorite?"), and to you and Mark Winterton for creating the world's most amazing kids.

Kate, my favorite girl, you inspire me with your smarts, courage, and independence. I wish I had half as much of all three when I was your age. You are amazing and a full-on joy to be around.

Andrew, my little pal and fellow Aries, I love every minute we spend together and smile for days afterward thinking about our adventures. Just please don't take me on a flight simulator ever again.

To my dad, Don Krikorian, a Renaissance man, whose little life lessons could fill a book. Thank you for your sense of humor, sharing with me your joy of cooking, and a lifetime of support. Thanks…for it all.

Sure, they call me a mama's girl, but I don't care. To the strong, witty, inspiring, and unwaveringly supportive Julia Krikorian: Every human on earth should be lucky enough to feel the kind of love you give. It keeps me smiling and fuels my days.

ABOUT THE AUTHOR

Stephanie Krikorian is a *New York Times* bestselling ghostwriter who has collaborated on more than twenty nonfiction books for various authors. Her widely read column, Hamptonomics, appears in the *New York Post*. Stephanie's work has also appeared in multiple publications including *O, the Oprah Magazine* and the *Wall Street Journal*, where she wrote about television and chronicled her second attempt at her first New York Marathon after her initial efforts were thwarted by Super Storm Sandy in 2012. She spent more than fifteen years in television news as a producer for CNBC and BusinessWeek TV. Stephanie also worked in digital news, developing and executive producing WSJ.com's live digital programming, and was the editor-in-charge of specials and planning for a digital news project at Reuters called Insider, which the *New York Times* referred to as "YouTube for traders." A reality television show that she created and executive produced was nominated for a New York Emmy. Stephanie graduated from the University of Western Ontario and has a Master of Science degree from Syracuse University's Newhouse School. She also studied wine at WSET, improv at the Upright Citizens Brigade, TV pilot and screenplay writing at the Writers' Program at UCLA Extension, and personal essay writing at both New York University and Columbia University. When she's not at the keyboard, she can be found in the yoga studio, on the farm picking vegetables, or on her paddleboard. Born and raised in Canada, Stephanie splits her time between New York City and East Hampton. *Zen Bender* is Stephanie's first solo book.